FIRST

The Nurse's Guide to Labs: A Quick and Easy Resource

BY CHERYL MILLER, EdD, MSN, RN

Professor of Nursing

Chattanooga State Community College

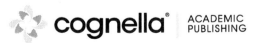 ACADEMIC PUBLISHING

Bassim Hamadeh, CEO and Publisher
Michael Simpson, Vice President, Acquisitions and Sales
Jamie Giganti, Senior Managing Editor
Miguel Macias, Graphic Designer
Angela Schultz, Senior Field Acquisitions Editor
Michelle Piehl, Project Editor
Alexa Lucido, Licensing Coordinator
Christian Berk, Associate Editor
Allie Kiekhofer, Interior Designer

Printed in the United States of America

ISBN: 978-1-5165-0098-7 (pbk) / 978-1-5165-0099-4 (br)

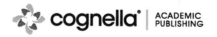

Contents

INTRODUCTION

This is a book about common lab tests and implications and application for nurses. The book is based on my knowledge and experience in teaching nursing students for over 30 years. Essentially, I am sharing my notes with you. Please feel free to add your notes as you gain experience in the clinical setting in the coming years. In fact, extra pages have been provided at the end for you to do so. It is my hope that this book will be a quick resource for you for years to come.

I got the idea for this book while teaching hematology to senior nursing students. The content covered many lab tests, and I continued to be amazed by the same comment that was made by students almost every year: "I wish I had known this earlier." I had assumed my lab content would be mainly a review for the students, but this was not so. For several semesters, the students had been completing lab data for their clients in clinical as they completed their care plans. However, I came to the conclusion that apparently they had not made the connections about the significance of the various lab tests as they completed their written assignments. Therefore, this is the purpose of this booklet.

As mentioned previously, this book is based on my general knowledge and experience. I will, however, be using a lab book titled *Davis's Comprehensive Handbook of Laboratory and Diagnostic Tests with Nursing Implications* written by

Anne M. Van Leeuwen and Mickey Lynn Bladh as my main reference book for lab values. This is the reference book currently used by my students.

Consider my book as merely a starting point for you. However, I hope it does cover most of the common lab tests you will see ordered for your clients. It is not intended to replace your more detailed reference lab book. You will still need to use additional resources. This book only covers adult clients, as values differ greatly with children of various ages. Values may be different for children, but the implications and application principles many times will be the same. The book also discusses mainly labs for adult clients in a medical-surgical setting and not those in the various specialty areas.

The book uses the following format for each lab test:

1. Definition (description of lab test—some pathology may be discussed)
2. The normal result
3. Critical result (if applicable)
4. Some common reasons for abnormal values
5. Nursing implications and responsibilities (this will include general nursing information, special preparation for the test, if any, and special care following the test, if any)

My goal is for you to become organized in your thinking and to see how fitting pieces of a puzzle together—by looking at lab values and all other assessment data—helps the health-care provider deliver the best possible care for clients. Lab values do not offer absolutes

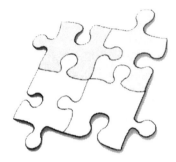

Figure 0-1 Jigsaw

in most situations. It is up to the clinician to decipher how pieces of the puzzle apply and what they mean.

There is one more piece of information for you before we get started. I want you to realize that "normal" lab values may vary slightly from hospital to hospital. Your facility's lab will define what is normal and abnormal. Again, as with children, the application and principles will remain basically the same once you determine that the value is abnormal. Once again, my reference (because we have to have a reference point) will be the book by Leeuwen and Bladh (2015).

Set your watch to go, and let's get started!

Image credit

- Fig. 0.1: https://commons.wikimedia.org/wiki/File%3AJigsaw.png. Copyright in the Public Domain.

OBJECTIVES

After reading this book, you should be able to:

1. Describe common lab tests ordered for the adult client in a medical-surgical setting.
2. Differentiate between normal and abnormal results.
3. Recognize abnormal values that are critical and require immediate action.
4. State some of the reasons for abnormal values.
5. Discuss various nursing implications and responsibilities when caring for a client ordered to have specific lab tests.
6. Understand the nursing implications and responsibilities when caring for a client with abnormal lab results.

1

LAB TESTS THAT ARE ORDERED COMBINED

Let's begin by discussing four groupings of labs that may be the first ones you ever see ordered for your clients. These help the health-care provider identify basic issues or perhaps validate assessment findings. They usually are ordered as a group because it is more cost effective than ordering the labs separately. These lab groupings are as follows:

1. Complete Blood Count (CBC)
2. Complete Blood Count with Differential
3. Basic Metabolic Panel
4. Complete Metabolic Panel

And now, let us begin our journey into the world of labs!

Complete Blood Count (CBC)

This is the most common lab test ordered. It is usually ordered to get a basic overview of the client's health/illness status. The lab is made up of the following components:

1. Hemoglobin (HGB)*
2. Hematocrit (HCT)*
3. Red Blood Cells (RBCs)
4. Mean Corpuscular Volume (MCV)
5. Mean Corpuscular Hemoglobin (MCH)
6. Mean Corpuscular Hemoglobin Concentration (MCHC)
7. Red Cell Distribution Width (RDW)
8. White Blood Cells (WBCs)*
9. Platelets (PLT)*
10. Mean Platelet Volume (MPV)

As the patient's nurse, you always should be aware of your patient's lab values for the items with an asterisk (*). You should always know four out of the ten items—that's not TOO hard!

Why should you know these? Each lab test will be discussed next individually.

Hemoglobin (HGB)*

Definition/Description

Hemoglobin is the molecule found on red blood cells that carries oxygen to the various body cells and transports CO_2 back to the lungs.

Normal Result

The normal result varies with age and gender. Why? It has a lot to do with hormonal levels, especially testosterone.

For the adult male, normal HGB is: 13.2–17.3 g/dL.

For the adult female, normal HGB is: 11.7–16.1 g/dL.

For the older adult male, normal HGB is: 12.6–17.4 g/dL.

For the older adult female, normal HGB is: 11.7–16.1 g/dL.

Critical Abnormal Result

Less than 6.6 g/dL

Greater than 20 g/dL

Some Common Reasons for Abnormalities

Decreased:

Various types of anemias (which will be discussed later—see MCV and MCHC)

Increased:

Erythrocytosis (Polycythemia vera is the most common type of erythrocytosis.)

Nursing Implications/Responsibilities

One action that the nurse should take first when a client's HGB report shows low or high is to look at other lab results to make sure the abnormality is not due to dehydration or overhydration. An HGB report can show high results with dehydration and low results with overhydration. If this is occurring, most likely the sodium (Na) and perhaps the Blood Urea Nitrogen (BUN) will show the same trend. Most importantly, the clinician should look at the history of the client and results obtained from the assessment.

If the HGB is truly low, the nurse must be prepared to implement all interventions appropriate for impaired activity intolerance. The nurse also must monitor oxygenation status of the client (pO_2 O_2 saturation, and respiratory rate). If the HGB is critically low, the nurse must be prepared to administer a blood transfusion, probably packed RBCs, if ordered.

If the HGB is increased, this can cause the blood to become sticky and viscous. This makes the heart have to work harder and could cause congestive heart failure over time. A high HBG also sets the patient up to be at risk for thrombus formation.

TIP: Remember, high altitudes and smoking can cause a client to have chronically high HGB. Both cause hypoxia, and the body tries to compensate by increasing HBG. Remember, you need to look at the entire picture!

Hematocrit (HCT)*

Definition/Description

Hematocrit represents the proportion of total blood volume that is made up of red blood cells. The lab value is expressed as a percentage. HGB and HCT go hand in hand, and if one is high or low, the same is true of the other. The purpose of this lab is to check for anemia or polycythemia. Hydration status also can be monitored. An increase in the hematocrit could mean dehydration, and a decrease could mean overhydration.

Normal Result

This varies according to age and gender, just like the hemoglobin results did.
Adult male: 38–51%
Adult female: 33–45%
Older male: 36–52%
Older female: 34–46%

Critical Abnormal Result

Less than 19.8%
Greater than 60%

Some Reasons for Abnormalities

Same as for HGB

Same as for HGB

TIP: HCT can be roughly calculated by taking the HGB value and multiplying it by 3. Example: If the HGB is 12, you can estimate that the HCT should be roughly 36%. However, this is true only if the red blood cells are normal in size and shape.

Red Blood Cells (RBCs)

Definition/Description

This lab determines the number of red blood cells per cubic millimeter of whole blood. Remember RBC production is regulated by the hormone, erythropoietin, from the kidneys. Red blood cells must have vitamin B12, folic acid, and iron for adequate production. RBCs normally live for 120 days and are destroyed by the spleen and converted to bilirubin in the liver. This lab is performed to mainly check for anemia or polycythemia. Low RBCs also could indicate certain kinds of cancers or kidney problems (remember the function of the kidneys and erythropoietin). HGB, HCT, and RBCs go hand in hand. Usually they go up or down together. The RBC count multiplied by 3 should approximate the HGB. (It has already been discussed that the HGB can be multiplied by 3 to obtain the approximate result of the HCT). Therefore, can you see how these three go hand in hand?

Normal Results

Normal results will vary according to gender and age.

Adult male: 5.21–5.81 × 10^6 cells/microL
Adult female: 3.91–5.11 × 10^6 cells/microL
Older male: 3.81–5.81 × 10^6 cells/microL
Older female: 3.71–5.31 × 10^6 cells/microL

The presence of any abnormally shaped cells such as those in the hemolytic anemia known as sickle cell anemia.

Various types of anemias
Hemorrhage
Cancer
Kidney problems
Overhydration

Polycythemia
Dehydration

Be prepared to administer blood products if ordered.

If anemia, implement nursing strategies for activity intolerance. If aplastic anemia is suspected, prepare to assist with bone marrow aspiration if ordered. If hemolytic anemia is suspected, be aware of bilirubin levels.

If polycythemia vera is present, prepare to assist with phlebotomy and implement strategies to prevent clotting.

Mean Corpuscular Volume (MCV)

This lab measures the average size of the red blood cells. It is useful in anemic conditions to help determine what type of anemia the client has. The size of

the red blood cell is denoted by the suffix-*cytic*. Red blood cells ca
sified as microcytic (small), normacytic (normal size), or macrocytic (large).
If they are microcytic, the MCV will be decreased; if normacytic, the MCV
will be a normal result; and if they are macrocytic, the MCV will be elevated.

Adult male: 77–97 (fL)
Adult female: 78–98 (fL)
Older adult male: 79–103 (fL)
Older adult female: 78–102 (fL)

N/A

Iron-deficiency anemia and thalassemia are examples of anemias that are
microcytic.

Aplastic anemia and blood loss are examples of anemias that are normacytic.
Pernicious anemia, vitamin B12 deficiency, folic acid deficiency, and alcoholism are examples of causes of anemias that are macrocytic.

Nothing specific other than interventions for anemia.

Mean Corpuscular Hemoglobin (MCH)

This lab measures the average amount of HGB on RBCs. It is used in helping
to diagnose the various types of anemias.

Adult male and female: 26–34 pg/cell
Older adult male and female: 27–35 pg/cell

N/A

Macrocytic anemias

Hypochromic anemias and microcytic anemias (The term, "hypochromic" is discussed next under MCHC)

Nothing specific other than interventions for anemia.

Mean Corpuscular Hemoglobin Concentration (MCHC)

This lab determines the average amount of HGB **per volume** of RBCs. It is done to assist in diagnosing various types of anemias. If the amount of hemoglobin is low in the volume of RBCs, the MCHC will be low and will be labeled as being hypochromic. If the amount of hemoglobin is normal in the volume of RBCs, the MCHC will be within normal limits and will be labeled as being normochromic. If the amount of hemoglobin is increased in the volume of RBCs, the MCHC will be increased and will be labeled as being hyperchromic.

32–36 g/dL

N/A

Decreased

Iron-deficiency anemia
Thalassemia

Nothing specific other than interventions for anemia.

Red Cell Distribution Width (RDW)

Definition/Description

This is a lab that measures the difference between the largest red blood cells and the smallest red blood cells. It is a measure of the variation between the two extremes. The health-care provider uses it to help differentiate between the various types of anemias.

Normal Result

11.6–14.8

Critical Abnormal Result

N/A

Various types of anemias will present with altered red cell distribution width. Do you realize there are over 400 different types of anemias?

Nursing Implications/Responsibilities

Nothing specific other than interventions for anemia.

White Blood Cells (WBCs)*

Definition/Description

The WBC count confirms the degree of response to a pathological condition and whether or not such a condition is present. WBCs are monitored to evaluate for the presence of infections. An increased WBC count can indicate an infection. The WBC count helps to give direction in determining a bacterial or viral infection. This lab also helps denote the inflammatory process and aids in the diagnosis of leukemias, lymphomas, and various neutropenic conditions. An increased WBC count is termed leukocytosis, while a decreased count is termed leukopenia.

Normal Result

$4.5–11.1 \times 10^3$/microL (4500–11,100/microL)

Critical Abnormal Results

Less than 2×10^3/microL (less than 2000/microL)
Greater than 30×10^3/microL (greater than 30,000/microL)

Some Common Reasons for Abnormalities

Decreased:
Bone marrow depression (such as aplastic anemia, toxic and antineoplastic drugs, or radiation)
Viral infections

Bacterial infections

Inflammatory process

Leukemias

Lymphomas

Polycythemia vera

Parasitic infection

Appendicitis

Nursing Implications/Responsibilities

If the WBC count is abnormal, the heath-care provider probably will order a differential to obtain more clues as to the cause of the abnormality. See WBC differential listed under Complete Blood Count with Differential.

Platelets (PLTs)*

Definition/Description

Platelets are small cell fragments in the blood that are formed in the bone marrow. They are necessary in adequate numbers for blood clotting. A deficiency in platelets is known as thrombocytopenia; an excess is known as thrombocytosis.

Normal Result

150,000–450,000/microL

Critical Abnormal Result

Less than 30,000/microL

Greater than 1,000,000/microL

Decreased:

Aplastic anemic

Medications

Immune mediated: examples of this are thrombocytopenic idiopathic purpura and heparin-induced thrombocytopenia (HIT)

DIC

Increased:

Splenectomy. This is because platelets are made in the bone marrow but stored in the spleen. With no spleen, platelets have no home; therefore, they must circulate in the vascular system.

Various types of cancers are associated with thrombocytosis. In fact, cancer must be ruled out with an increased platelet result with no obvious rationale for the increased amount.

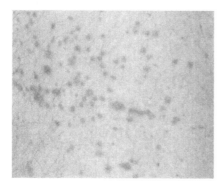

Figure 1-1 Purpura

Nursing Implications/ Responsibilities

If available, the nurse should always monitor the client's platelet level. If decreased to a critical level, the nurse must initiate bleeding precautions. Any client with a platelet level of less than 30,000/microL should remain on bed rest in order to decrease the risk for falls. Platelets will be ordered to be administered. Platelets do not have to be typed and cross matched. They arrive frozen and must be thawed before administration. Sometimes, several units of platelets have to be administered.

If the nurse observes purpura or petechiae on a client, platelet count should be reviewed immediately.

At a level of around 60,000/microL, clients can bleed excessively with trauma.
At a level of around 20,000/microL, clients can bleed spontaneously without trauma.
Bleeding into the brain is a special concern.

At a level of 1,000,000/microL, clients can have a tendency to form thrombi because of the crowding of platelets. However, they can also bleed because since platelets are being produced at such a rapid rate, they do not have time to mature and be effective.

Mean Platelet Volume (MPV)

Definition/Description

This lab test determines the average size of platelets. Younger platelets are generally larger in size. An increase in this lab (MPV) indicates an increase in platelet turnover. They are either being destroyed too early or something is occurring to cause increased production of platelets.

Normal Result

7.1–10.2 (fL)

Critical Abnormal Result

N/A

Some Common Reasons for Abnormalities

Low MPV can be suspicious for toxic drugs.
High MPV with low platelet count is suspicious for immune-induced thrombocytopenia.

High MPV with normal platelet count can be a sign of chronic myeloid leukemia.
High MPV can help support a diagnosis of aplastic anemia (with other supporting data).

Education: A high MPV indicates a high tendency for clotting, therefore increasing a client's risk for stroke and cardiac problems. It is usually important that the health-care provider order prophylactic aspirin for this client.

Education: A low MPV indicates a greater bleeding risk especially with a low platelet count. This client should be taught bleeding precautions and aspirin precautions.

Complete Blood Count with Differential

This lab group consists of all of the components of the complete blood count (CBC). It is different from the CBC in that it also includes a breakdown of the types of white blood cells. This is usually ordered when the WBCs are abnormal, and the health-care provider needs to look for clues as to why the WBCs are abnormal. It is important for you, the nurse, to know the results of the WBC differential.

The differential component of the CBC includes the breakdown of the following white blood cells:

1. Granulocytes
    a. Neutrophils
    b. Eosinophils
    c. Basophils

2. Agranulocytes
    a. Lymphocytes
    b. Monocytes

Each of these will be discussed separately on the following pages.

Neutrophils

Definition/Description

Neutrophils are the immune's system first line of defense against the inflammatory process or an infection, usually a bacterial infection. They act through phagocytosis and contain substances that can combat foreign invaders. They are the most abundant of all of the white blood cells in normal healthy conditions.

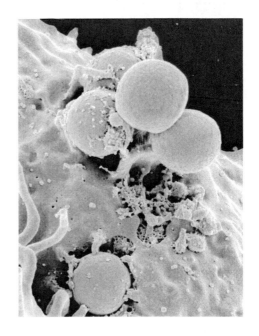

They are sometimes called poly morphonuclear cells and can also be called segmented neutrophils. Immature neutrophils are called bands. "Baby" or immature neutrophils (bands) usually are not found in abundance in the circulating blood and, at the most, account for 3–5% of total white blood cells in healthy conditions. During the infectious process, bands may increase

Figure 1-2 Human neutrophil ingesting MRSA

significantly. This shows that the immune system is trying to work overtime to send out neutrophils from the bone marrow. However, the bone marrow does not have time to let the neutrophils mature. "Babies" cannot do the work of grown-ups!

This whole process of increased bands sometimes is referred to as a "shift to the left" and indicates an infectious process. You should consider pneumonia if bands increase to greater than 12% of the total white blood cell count and perhaps consider sepsis with a band count of greater than 20%.

Normal Result

40–75% of total white blood cell count

Critical Abnormal Result

Absolute neutrophil count (ANC) of less than 0.5×10^{3}/microL (see below)

Some Common Reasons for Abnormalities

Decreased:
Viral infections
Toxic and antineoplastic drugs (chemotherapy)
Radiation
Malnutrition
Any condition that alters the immune system
Aplastic anemia

Increased:
Infections—particularly bacterial
Inflammatory response
Malignancies
Stress
Steroid use

Nursing Implications/Responsibilities

The absolute neutrophil count (ANC) is used to help assess a person's immune status. It often is used during chemotherapy to determine if a client's immune status is sufficient for additional chemotherapy. Remember, chemotherapy suppresses a person's immune system even more!

ANC is calculated in the following way:
ANC = Total WBC × (% segmented neutrophils + % of bands)
Example: If the total WBC is 5,000 and the segs are 40% and the bands are 5%, the ANC is calculated as: 5,000 × (0.40 + 0.05) = 5,000 × .45 = 2,250

1500 or above generally is okay.

Mild neutropenia exists with a count of 1000–1500.

Moderate neutropenia exists with a count of 500–1000.

Severe neutropenia exists with a count of less than 500.

The ANC also has implications for the nurse in deciding when to place a client on reverse isolation precautions for suppressed immunity.

Eosinophils

Definition/Description

An increase in this type of white blood cell could indicate some type of parasitic infection or some type of allergic reaction.

Normal Result

0–5.5% of the total white blood cell count

Critical Abnormal Result

N/A

Some Common Reasons for Abnormalities

Decreased:

Aplastic anemia

Stress

Increased:

Parasitic infection

Allergy

Asthma

Dermatitis

Eczema

Hay fever

Remember, if one type of white blood cell goes up, another type has to decrease. The total white blood cell count is a percentage, so 100% is the maximum. The bone marrow adjusts.

Basophils

Definition/Description

Basophils usually make up a small percentage of white blood cells. They contain histamine and serotonin. When these white blood cells migrate to the lungs, they are called mast cells. They can increase during allergic conditions as they release histamine and cause some of the signs and symptoms seen in allergic reactions and in anaphylactic reactions.

Normal Result

0–1%

Critical Abnormal Result

N/A

Some Common Reasons for Abnormalities

Increased:

Hypersensitivity states

Nursing Implications/Responsibilities

Nurses usually think of elevated basophils as being associated with respiratory symptoms and hypersensitivities. While this is certainly true, elevated basophils also can be associated with other conditions such as leukemia, Hodgkin's disease, ulcerative colitis, and polycythemia vera.

Lymphocytes

These cells are part of the agranulocytes and are the second most abundant white blood cells in healthy conditions. Lymphocytes are divided into two basic types—B cells and T cells. Both are formed in the bone marrow. B cells mature in the bone marrow, but T cells have to travel to the thymus gland for maturation. T lymphocytes are involved with cell-mediated immunity. B cells are involved with antigen recognition and antibody formation. T cells consist of helper cells, killer cells, and suppressor cells. The helper T cell is the "quarterback" of the immune system. It recognizes foreign antigens and turns the immune system on. This is the cell that is destroyed with HIV/AIDS. The person with HIV/AIDS loses the "quarterback," and thus the result is the development of various opportunistic infections.

Normal Result

12–44% of the total white blood cell count

Critical Abnormal Result

N/A

Some Common Reasons for Abnormalities

Decreased:
HIV/AIDS
Other immunodeficiency diseases
Adrenocorticosteroids
Antineoplastic drugs
Radiation
Aplastic anemia
Bone marrow failure
Stress

Viral infections

Lymphocytic leukemia

Lymphomas

Thyrotoxicosis

Infectious mononucleosis

Nursing Implications/Responsibilities

The nurse should be aware that the lymphocyte count can be decreased very rapidly after X-ray treatment or after large doses of vitamins such as niacin and thiamine!

Monocytes

Definition/Description

These cells are agranulocytes but closely related to neutrophils as far as function. These cells have the major role of phagocytosis. They help other cells remove damaged tissue and thus stop the inflammatory process. They also are fighters and protect against bacteria, viruses, and fungi.

Normal Result

4–9 % of the total white blood cell count

Critical Abnormal Result

N/A

Some Common Reasons for Abnormalities

Increased:

Active tuberculosis

End of infection or inflammatory process (see below)

During an infection or inflammatory process, if neutrophils start to decrease and monocytes start to increase, this could be an indicator that the infection/inflammation is improving or subsiding.

Basic Metabolic Panel (BMP)

The basic metabolic panel is a group of labs that may be ordered along with the CBC. The purpose is to give the health-care provider an overview of the health status of the client. These tests are ordered together because it is more cost effective than to order them separately. Usually, it is preferred that this group of labs be done while the patient is fasting, although this is not always possible. The tests that make up the basic metabolic panel are as follows:

1. BUN (Blood Urea Nitrogen)
2. Calcium
3. Chloride
4. CO_2
5. Creatinine (serum)
6. Glucose
7. Potassium
8. Sodium

Each of these will be discussed individually on the following pages.

Blood Urea Nitrogen (BUN)

Definition/Description

This lab measures the amount of urea nitrogen in the blood. Urea nitrogen is the product of protein metabolism. It is formed from ammonia in the liver and then has to be excreted in the kidneys. Basically, the BUN is an expression of the balance between protein intake and protein excretion. Since kidneys are very involved with this entire process, the BUN often is reviewed with the creatinine. In fact, for the "balance" to be "intact," the BUN/creatinine ratio should be 15:1–24:1. See below for a detailed explanation.

Normal Result

Adult: 8–21 mg/dL
Adult > 90 years of age: 10–31 mg/dL
BUN/Creatinine Ratio: 15:1–24:1

Critical Abnormal Result

Greater than 100 mg/dL (non-dialysis patients)

Some Common Reasons for Abnormalities

Decreased:
Low-protein diet
Malnutrition
Overhydration
Liver failure

Increased:
Kidney disease
High-protein intake
GI bleeding (protein of cell walls being broken down)
Urinary tract blockage
Burns
Dehydration

Nursing Implications/Responsibilities

BUN and creatinine go together like bread and butter. However, an increased BUN does not always mean kidney dysfunction. You must look at the BUN/ creatinine ratio! If both BUN and creatinine are increased, the ratio will most likely be normal (within the 15:1–24:1 ratio), and this most likely indicates some type of kidney dysfunction. If only the BUN is increased, the ratio will be increased, and this indicates a non-kidney problem is causing the increase in the BUN.

The BUN/creatinine ratio is determined by dividing the BUN result by the creatinine result. The answer is the number other than 1 that you are looking for in the ratio—normal should be between 15 and 24.
Wow—this is getting difficult and confusing, so let's look at two examples!

Example #1
BUN: 55 mg/dL
Creatinine: 2.3 mg/dL
Ratio is calculated by: 55/2.3 = 23.9
The 23.9 is between the normal value of 15 and 24, so the ratio is normal. However, both the creatinine and the BUN are increased, so the conclusion is that this is probably a kidney dysfunction.

Example #2
BUN: 55 mg/dL
Creatinine: 0.8 mg/dL
Ratio is calculated by: 55/0.8 = 68.75
The 68.75 is NOT between the normal ratio of 15 and 24. The BUN is the only result that is elevated; the creatinine is within normal limits. The conclusion is that the elevation of the BUN is due to a non-kidney reason.

Calcium (Ca)

Definition/Description

Calcium is mainly stored in the teeth and bones. There is a smaller amount found in the blood. The calcium in the blood is either bound to albumin or unbound, where it is known as ionized calcium.

The calcium in the blood can be measured by two different methods. Total serum calcium includes both bound and unbound calcium. Ionized calcium measures only the unbound calcium. Ionized calcium may be more accurate, especially if the albumin level is low. Therefore, if the total serum calcium is abnormal, the health-care provider may order an ionized calcium to clarify that the calcium is truly abnormal.

Another important point to remember about calcium is that is works in a reverse relationship with phosphorus. If serum calcium is elevated, serum phosphorus will be decreased. All of this works under the control of the parathyroid hormone. Remember, the parathyroid hormone needs vitamin D to function effectively.

Normal Result

Total Serum Calcium
Adult: 8.2–10.2 mg/dL
Adult older than 90 years old: 8.2–9.6 mg/dL

Ionized Calcium
4.64–5.28 mg/dL

Critical Abnormal Result

Total Serum Calcium
Less than 7 mg/dL
Greater than 12 mg/dL

Ionized Calcium
Less than 3.2mg/dL
Greater than 6.2 mg/dL

Some Common Reasons for Abnormalities

Decreased:
High phosphate levels
Kidney disease
Removal of parathyroid gland
Thyroidectomy (with accidental removal of parathyroid glands)
Vitamin D deficiency

Certain cancers
Parathyroid gland disorders
Bone diseases
Prolonged bed rest
Parathyroid tumor

Nursing Implications/Responsibilities

High Calcium

The nurse should always think of stones! Strain all urine. Get patient out of bed if possible (bed rest causes loss of calcium from bones and makes serum calcium go even higher). Bones may be brittle, though, since calcium goes from bones to blood while the patient is on bed rest. Therefore precautions will need to be taken to prevent falls while patient is out of bed.

High calcium can also cause personality changes in clients—some may appear as though they have Alzheimer's, and some may even appear psychotic!

For treating high calcium, always think of hydration—hydration—and more hydration—IV at a fast rate, if possible. Probably normal saline will be the fluid of choice since it is an isotonic solution and will stay in the vascular space. Diuretics can be given along with phosphate. Dialysis may be a last resort.

Low Calcium

The nurse should watch for tetany. The main problem associated with tetany is airway obstruction. Tetany causes constriction and contractions of the airway and larynx—can be fatal!! Remember the warning signs of low calcium: numbness and tingling. Review Chvostek's sign and Trousseau's sign so you can be aware if the patient exhibits signs and symptoms associated with these!

Low calcium can be treated with calcium. There are two main types that are used—calcium chloride and calcium gluconate. Keep in mind that calcium chloride is more concentrated. It contains 270 mg of calcium per gram while calcium gluconate contains 90 mg.

Any time a patient receives calcium IV, he or she should be on a cardiac monitor.

TIP: To help myself remember the entire calcium and phosphorus relationship, I relate it to kidney disease and what happens in that scenario.

1. The kidneys fail.
2. Phosphorus must be excreted by kidneys, but in kidney failure, this does not happen.
3. Phosphorus levels increase in the blood.
4. An increased phosphorus level in the blood causes the serum calcium to decrease because calcitonin from the thyroid pushes the calcium back into the bones.
5. Low serum calcium stimulates the parathyroid gland to secrete parathyroid hormone.
6. This hormone pulls calcium from the bones and teeth to try to raise serum calcium.
7. Cycle continues—this is why a client in kidney failure has increased phosphorus, decreased calcium, increased parathyroid hormone, and brittle bones!

Chloride (Cl)

Definition/Description

This is a lab that helps with giving the health-care provider a quick look to see if there could be a problem with hydration, electrolytes, or acid-base balance.

Chloride is a negatively charged ion (anion). It is the most abundant anion in the blood. It competes with bicarbonate (another anion) for sodium (Na+) (a positive ion is called a cation). This is how chloride helps in controlling acid/base balance; remember the importance of bicarbonate in acid/base balance.

Chloride also helps with water balance because it usually follows Na+ unless some other type of problem is occurring.

One of the reasons chloride is included in the basic metabolic panel is so the health-care provider can detect any unmeasured anions. This can be done by calculation of the anion gap, which is done as follows:

$Na^+ + K^+$ minus $Cl^- + HCO_3^-$

A normal anion gap is less than 11 mEq/L. Any result above that indicates that a closer look should be taken into electrolytes, hydration, and/or acid-base balance.

Normal Result

97–107 mEq/L

Critical Abnormal Result

Less than 80 mEq/L
Greater than 115 mEq/L

Some Common Reasons for Abnormalities

Decreased:

Addison's disease: (chloride follows Na)
Burns (chloride follows Na)
Heart failure (dilutional)
Excessive sweating (loss)
Vomiting (loss)
Overhydration (dilutional)

Increased:

Renal failure (cannot eliminate)
Cushing's disease (chloride follows Na)
Dehydration (concentration)
Diabetes insipidus (concentration)
Normal saline infusion (intake)
Acid/base imbalance

Signs and symptoms of hypochloremia are as follows: tremors, twitching, shallow breathing, and decreased blood pressure.

Signs and symptoms of hyperchloremia are as follows: weakness, lethargy, and deep rapid breathing.

However, usually the health-care provider does not look for these specific signs and symptoms because if chloride levels are abnormal, there will be other electrolyte imbalances or acid/base imbalances that have more dominant signs and symptoms.

CO_2

Definition/Description

This lab is used to assess acid-base balance and helps to let the health-care provider know if acid/base problems could exist. CO_2 in this lab stands for CO_2 content, and it exists in the blood mainly as bicarbonate (HCO_3). This represents the first buffer component in regulating acid/base balance. This is NOT the same as pCO_2 in an arterial blood gas, which is thought of as acidic. It gets confusing because in this lab, CO_2 needs to be thought of as an alkaline because 95% of CO_2 is bound in venous blood as bicarbonate (HCO_3). This is the second largest anion found in the blood, the first being chloride.

Normal Result

Whole Blood: Venous Blood
22–26 mEq/L or mmol/L

Critical Abnormal Result

Less than 15 mEq/L or mmol/L
Greater than 40 mEq/L or mmol/L

"Interpretation requires clinical information and evaluation of other electrolytes" (Van Leeuwen & Bladh, 2015, p. 367).
Vomiting or gastric suctioning can cause increased CO_2 levels.

Nursing Implications/Responsibilities

Specimen needs to be stored under anaerobic conditions to prevent the diffusion of CO_2 from the specimen.

Creatinine (Serum)

Definition/Description

This lab is done for the purpose of checking kidney function.

Creatinine is a waste product from energy being supplied to muscles and other tissues. It only can be removed from the blood by the kidneys. Therefore, if kidney failure is present, the creatinine will be elevated. Sometimes this lab is ordered with the blood urea nitrogen (BUN) for comparison. The BUN/creatinine ratio should be 15:1–24:1. Most times, an estimate will be calculated with the creatinine to see how fast the kidneys are clearing creatinine from the blood. This is known as the estimated glomerular filtration rate (eGFR). Refer to GFR under the renal section of this book for more detailed information.

Normal Result

Normal result varies according to gender.
Adult male: 0.61–1.21 mg/dL
Adult female: 0.51–1.11 mg/dL
Note: Creatinine generally decreases as people age because of loss of muscle mass.

Greater than 7.4 mg/dL (for a client NOT on dialysis)

Decreased muscle mass
Hyperthyroidism (increased GFR)

Renal disease: acute and chronic
Renal calculi (decreased excretion)
Rhabdomyolysis
Acromegaly/gigantism (increased muscle mass)

Chronic renal insufficiency is suspected with creatinine levels between 1.5 and 3.0 mg/dL.

Chronic renal failure is suspected with creatinine levels greater than 3.0 mg/dL.

Glucose

The most common purpose of this lab is to assess for diabetes. It also can be used to evaluate disorders of carbohydrate metabolism. Other uses are to help identify hypoglycemia and to monitor the effectiveness of medications.

Fasting: Less than 100 mg/dL

Less than 40 mg/dL
Greater than 400 mg/dL

Some Common Reasons for Abnormalities

Decreased:

Addison's disease
Starvation
Glycogen storage diseases
Hypothyroidism

Increased:

Diabetes
Acromegaly/gigantism
Stress
Cushing's disease
Pancreatitis
Pheochromocytoma
Thyrotoxicosis

Nursing Implications/Responsibilities

"The American Diabetes Association and National Institute of Diabetes and Digestive and Kidney Diseases consider a confirmed fasting blood glucose greater than 126 mg/dL to be consistent with a diagnosis of diabetes" (Van Leeuwen & Bladh, 2015, 854).

The test for glucose is one of the main reasons the BMP should be done when the patient has fasted at least eight hours. Health-care provider should be notified if the result is NOT a fasting glucose.

WHY IS IT IMPORTANT FOR THE NURSE TO KNOW THE CLIENT'S GLUCOSE LEVEL?

At glucose levels around 30 mg/dL, a client can have seizures.

At glucose levels around 20 mg/dL, a client can have irreversible brain damage.

Potassium (K)

This lab is used to measure the quantity of K^+ since this electrolyte has many important functions in the body. It transmits electrical impulses to cardiac and skeletal muscle. It also assists in acid/base balance with the exchange of H^+ ions and K^+ ions in the renal tubules. It helps with fluid balance by its relationship with sodium. Generally, as potassium goes up, sodium goes down. Potassium is controlled by the release of aldosterone from the adrenal glands. Aldosterone causes sodium to be retained and potassium to be excreted by the kidneys.

This lab also is used to indirectly assess renal disease and monitor clients on digitalis therapy and diuretics.

Potassium is stored INSIDE of cells, so there is only a small amount in the blood.

Normal Result

3.5–5.3 mEq/L or mmol/L

Critical Abnormal Result

Less than 2.8 mEq/L or mmol/L
Greater than 6.2 mEq/L or mmol/L

Some Common Reasons for Abnormalities

Decreased:
Alkalosis
Cushing's disease
Inadequate intake
GI loss
Some diuretics
Overhydration

Acidosis

Acute renal failure

Addison's disease

Dehydration

Dialysis clients

Excessive use of salt substitutes

Transfusion of old banked blood

Insulin deficiency

Ketoacidosis

Early stage of burn injury

Nursing Implications/Responsibilities

The nurse must remember that potassium, in any form other than oral tablets, must be diluted. Tablets should not be crushed. Oral liquid should be diluted in water or orange juice. If given IV, it must be given at a certain concentration and at a slow rate.

Before potassium is given to a patient, make sure he or she has adequate kidney function and can void, as that is the only way excess potassium can be eliminated from the body.

Too much or too little potassium in the body can cause muscle problems—cardiac is the one that can cause the most serious problems.

Low potassium also is associated with muscle weakness and therefore falls.

Remember that pH and K^+ have an inverse relationship. As blood pH decreases (acidosis), K^+ levels tend to rise.

Sodium (Na)

Definition/Description

This lab test is used to monitor the quantity of sodium in the blood since this electrolyte has many very important functions in the body. It is involved with maintaining osmotic pressure of the extracellular fluid; it is involved in renal retention and excretion of water; it helps with maintaining acid/base balance; it helps maintain blood pressure; and it helps in the regulation of K^+.

Sodium is the most abundant cation in the extracellular fluid.
It is one of the first labs that the heath-care provider reviews to assess the hydration status of the client.

Normal Result

135–145 mEq/L or mmol/L

Critical Abnormal Result

Less than 120 mEq/L or mmol/L
Greater than 160 mEq/L or mmol/L

Some Common Reasons for Abnormalities

Decreased:
Heart failure (fluid retention and dilution)
Cystic fibrosis
SIADH (dilutional)
Diuretics
Addison's disease
Nephrotic syndrome

Increased:
Excessive water loss
Dehydration
Cushing's disease

Diabetes

Excessive intake

Hyperaldosteronism

Remember:

0.9% sodium chloride is isotonic (stays in the vascular space).

0.45% sodium chloride is hypotonic (moves out of the vascular space and into the cells).

3%–5% sodium chloride is hypertonic (moves from the cells back into the vascular space).

CAUTION: Hypertonic solutions must be given at the prescribed rate, which will be SLOW. Pulling fluid too rapidly from the cells can cause them to collapse and can be fatal to the client. An example of this is central pontine myelinolysis (CPM), where cells are destroyed in the brainstem.

Why Is It Important for the Nurse to Know the Client's Na⁺ Level?

With an Na⁺ level around 125 mEq/L, the client will start to become nauseated.

With an Na⁺ level around 115–120 mEq/L, the client will complain of a headache and start to become lethargic.

With an Na⁺ level around 110–115 mEq/L, the client will start to have seizures and slip into a coma.

Comprehensive Metabolic Panel (CMP)

The comprehensive metabolic panel contains all components of the basic metabolic panel. It also contains albumin, total protein, and the various liver labs. Again, it is generally more cost effective to order the tests as a group rather than ordering individual tests. The additional tests for this panel, besides the ones in the basic metabolic panel, are as follows:

1. Albumin
2. Total Protein
3. Alkaline Phosphatase (ALP)
4. Alanine Amino Transferase (ALT) (formerly called SGPT)
5. Aspartate Amino Transferase (AST) (formerly called SGOT)
6. Bilirubin

Each of the above labs will be discussed individually on the following pages.

Albumin

Definition/Description

This lab is used to check nutritional status for a client, mainly a chronic protein deficiency (prealbumin is more accurate in assessing for a short-term deficiency within the last 30 days). The lab also is used to check for liver or kidney disease. Albumin is made in the liver, and it should NOT be excreted unless there is some type of pathology within the kidneys. This lab also is used to evaluate fluid status, as a function of albumin is to hold water in the vascular space.

Albumin is normally the largest component of the total protein in the blood plasma. It is a transport protein, and as mentioned above, it affects plasma osmotic pressure, which regulates fluids between the vascular tree and the tissues.

Normal Result

Albumin levels decrease with age.
Adult 20–40 years of age: 3.7–5.1 g/dL
Adult 41–60 years of age: 3.4–4.8 g/dL
Adult 61–90 years of age: 3.2–4.6 g/dL
Adult >90 years of age: 2.9–4.5 g/dL

N/A

However, it is important to note the A/G ratio, where *A* stands for albumin and *G* stands for globulin. The formula for calculating the A/G ratio is as follows: Albumin/(total protein-albumin).

A ratio of less than 1.0, where globulin exceeds albumin, is significant clinically.

Example: A client has an albumin level of 3.7 g/dL and a total protein of 8 g/dL. The A/G ratio would be calculated as follows: 3.7/(8-3.7) = 3.7/4.3 = 0.86. This would be clinically significant.

Some Common Reasons for Abnormalities

Decreased:

Overhydration
Inefficient protein intake
Liver inefficiency (alcoholism, cirrhosis, etc.)
Burns
Hemorrhage
Kidney Disease
Pre-eclampsia
Enteropathies
Ulcerative colitis
Crohn's disease

Increased:

Dehydration
Hyper-infusion of albumin

Nursing Implications/Responsibilities

If dehydration or overhydration is suspected, the nurse should look at other lab results, which should be trending in the same direction such as HGB, HCT, and Na^+.

Total Protein

This lab is used to assess nutritional status and is also used to assess fluid status.

Total protein consists of albumin and all of the globulins—alpha, beta, and gamma globulins. Proteins are the building blocks for the body and are required for metabolic processes and maintaining water balance within the body. Albumin makes up the largest component of total protein in normal healthy situations.

Normal Result

6–8 g/dL

Critical Abnormal Result

N/A

Some Common Reasons for Abnormalities

Decreased:

Fluid excess (IV administration—due to hemodilution)
Burns (loss of protein through vascular walls)
Alcoholism (lack of protein intake)
Ulcerative colitis (lack of absorption)
Cirrhosis (liver cannot produce)
Crohn's disease (lack of absorption)
Glomerulonephritis (kidney permeability problems)
Heart failure (dilution)
Malnutrition (inadequate protein intake)

Increased:

Dehydration (due to concentration)
Myeloma (excessive production of gamma globulins)

Refer to the A/G ratio discussed with albumin.

Alkaline Phosphatase (ALP)

Definition/Description

This lab is used to help in the diagnosis of liver problems such as cancer or cirrhosis. It also helps in the diagnosis of bone cancer or bone fracture. How does this work? ALP is an enzyme found mainly in the liver, in Kupffer cells of the biliary tract, intestines, and in bones. The enzyme is named alkaline because it prefers places where a high pH exists.

Twelve isoenzymes of ALP have been identified. Three are clinically significant: ALP_1 of the liver, ALP_2 of the bones, and ALP_3 of the intestines.

Normal Result

Results vary according to a person's gender and age.

	ALP	ALP_1 Liver	ALP_2 Bone
Male 21 years and older	35–142 units/L	0–93 units/L	11–73 units/L
Female 21 years and older	25–125 units/L	0–93 units/L	11–73 units/L

Critical Abnormal Result

N/A

Decreased:

Anemia

HIV/AIDS

Nutritional deficiencies (especially of zinc and magnesium)

Increased:

Liver disease

Biliary obstruction

Cancer of the colon, gallbladder, lung, or pancreas

Healing fractures

Perforated bowel

Hepatitis

Nursing Implications/Responsibilities

There are no pretesting restrictions for this lab as far as food, fluids, or medications. However, if a client has been non-fasting and has consumed a fatty meal prior to the lab, a false elevation could occur. A fasting lab probably would be ordered at this point.

Alanine Amino Transferase (ALT)

Definition/Description

The purpose of this lab is to check for liver disease or liver damage. It is useful in monitoring for damage from hepatotoxic medications.

ALT is an enzyme produced by the liver when liver damage has occurred. ALT levels can increase up to 50 times the normal amount. The enzyme is found in smaller amounts in the kidney, heart, pancreas, spleen, skeletal muscles, and erythrocytes.

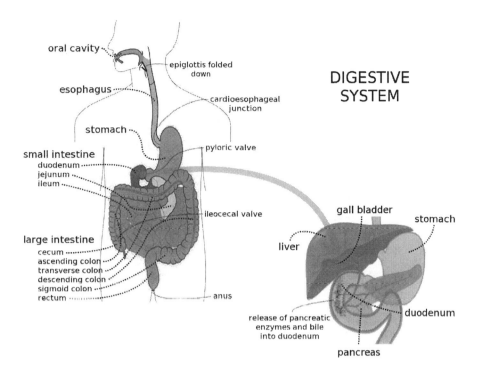

Figure 1-3 Digestive system with liver

Normal Result

Varies according to age and gender.

Young/middle-aged adult male: 10–40 units/L

Young/middle-aged adult female: 7–35 units/L

61–90-year-old male: 13–40 units/L

61–90-year-old female: 10–28 units/L

Greater than 90 years of age – male: 6–38 units/L

Greater than 90 years of age – female: 5–24 units/L

Critical Abnormal Result

N/A

Liver disease

Liver damage

Pancreatitis

Myocardial infarction

Burns

Acetaminophen overdose

Hepatitis

Nursing Implications/Responsibilities

One lab cannot determine liver dysfunction. This is one example where the clinician must look at a variety of labs to best determine how to proceed with care for that client. Each lab is only one piece of the puzzle we discussed at the beginning of this book.

Aspartate Amino Transferase (AST)

Definition/Description

The purpose of this lab is to assess for liver disease or liver damage. It also can be used to assess for myocardial infarction, although it is used to a lesser extent for that today. AST is an enzyme that is elevated in most liver disorders. It is elevated at the highest levels in conditions that are associated with necrosis such as viral hepatitis and cirrhosis.

Normal Result

Varies with age and gender.

20–49-year-old male: 20–40 units/L

20–49-year-old female: 15–30 units/L

Greater than 50-year-old male: 10–35 units/L

Greater than 45-year-old female: 10–35 units/L

N/A

Decreased:

Clients receiving hemodialysis (deficiency of vitamin B_6)

Increased:

Acute hepatitis (especially viral)
Drug overdoses
Acute pancreatitis
Alcohol abuse
Cirrhosis
Liver tumors

Nursing Implications/Responsibilities

Values > 500 units/L are usually associated with hepatitis, liver problems in acute stage, or drug toxicities in overdoses. The lab is elevated to a lesser extent with other liver problems.

Bilirubin

Definition/Description

The purpose of this lab is to check for diseases of the liver or diseases that can affect the liver directly.

The lab is a combination of total bilirubin, which is then broken down into unconjugated and conjugated bilirubin. When the total bilirubin result is abnormal, it is important to look at the values for unconjugated and conjugated bilirubin. By doing so, the health-care provider can have a better clue as to the source of the problem. Continue reading for the explanation for this!

Bilirubin is a breakdown product of destroyed red blood cells. Red blood cells are destroyed normally after 120 days in circulation. They are destroyed by the spleen. From the spleen, the destroyed cells are carried to the liver by albumin. At this point, before they reach the liver, they are classified as unconjugated bilirubin, or indirect bilirubin. In the liver, the indirect bilirubin goes through another process and becomes conjugated; the name then changes to conjugated, or direct, bilirubin.

With an abnormal total bilirubin value result, the health-care provider can get a better understanding of the source of the problem by looking at the lab report for the unconjugated and the conjugated bilirubin. If the unconjugated is abnormal, the problem lies before the liver; and if the conjugated bilirubin is more abnormal, the problem most likely lies within the liver.

Normal Result

Total bilirubin: Less than 1.2 mg/dL
Unconjugated bilirubin: Less than 1.1 mg/dL
Conjugated bilirubin: Less than 0.3 mg/dL

Critical Abnormal Result

Greater than 15 mg/dL
What happens with this high level?
Increased bilirubin is referred to as hyperbilirubinemia which can lead to brain damage if sustained over a period of time. Kernicterus is a term you should be familiar with because it is the term used when bilirubin is deposited in the brainstem and basal ganglia. Even though this is a book regarding adults, I cannot refrain from telling you that infants are at high risk for hyperbilirubinemia and the development of kernicterus. Look up the signs and symptoms so you will be prepared to care for your client no matter whether adult or infant as this is a serious condition.

Some Common Reasons for Abnormalities

Decreased:
N/A

Increased:

Unconjugated, or indirect, bilirubin:

Hemolytic anemias

Large hematomas

Conjugated or direct bilirubin:

Tumors of the liver

Biliary obstruction problems

Cirrhosis

Hepatitis

Nursing Implications/Responsibilities

The health-care provider may request that the client fast before the test. Bilirubin is light sensitive so the blood sample container must be kept covered. By knowing this, can you guess why bilirubin lights are a form of treatment for hyperbilirubinemia?

With increased bilirubin, the nurse will assess for jaundice (also called icterus). Jaundice shows up most readily on the client's skin and in the sclera of the eyes. However, bilirubin in the urine can be detected before jaundice appears.

Image credits

2 ADDITIONAL INDIVIDUAL ELECTROLYTES

Magnesium (Mg)

Definition/Description

Magnesium is usually stored in cells and bones and is the second most abundant intracellular cation. Its major role is to help sodium (Na^+) and potassium (K^+) move in and out of cells, as well as a variety of other functions involving energy, cells, and enzymatic processes. It also is needed for nerve transmission and to enable muscles to relax. Magnesium is the fourth most abundant cation overall.

Normal Result

1.6–2.6 mg/dL

Critical Abnormal Result

Greater than 4.9 mg/dL
Less than 1.2 mg/dL

Some Common Reasons for Abnormalities

Decreased:
Alcohol abuse
Starvation

Diuretics

Conditions that are associated with decreased calcium (decreased calcium and decreased magnesium usually occur together).

Taking too many antacids and/or laxatives containing magnesium
Kidney failure

Nursing Implications/Responsibilities

Excessive magnesium can cause neuromuscular and cardiac depression, with symptoms such as bradycardia, decreased reflexes, prolonged PR and/or QT interval, respiratory arrest, or cardiac arrest.

Toxic levels of magnesium can be reversed by administration of fluids and/or dialysis.

Decreased magnesium can cause ventricular tachycardia (especially torsades), tremors, and tetany.
Magnesium MUST be replaced.

Why Is It Important for the Nurse to Know the Client's Magnesium Level?

Other than all of the potential cardiac issues such as coding, seizures can occur with low magnesium levels!

Phosphorus (P)

Definition/Description

Phosphorus is used in the body for growing bones and teeth. It is also important for muscle contraction. It is found in the body as the phosphate ion and is the major intracellular anion; 85% is stored in bones, and the rest is found in cells and body fluids. Its release is under the control of the parathyroid gland and the kidneys.

2.5–4.5 mg/dL

Less than 1.0 mg/dL
Greater than 8.9 mg/dL

Decreased:
Hypercalcemia
Alcohol abuse
Poor nutrition

Increased:
Kidney disease
Bone disease
Bone metastases
Hypocalcemia
Low vitamin D levels
Low parathyroid hormone
Acidosis (pushes out of cells)

Nursing Implications/Responsibilities

Because phosphorus and calcium have an inverse relationship, if phosphorus is high, the patient with a minor increase could be ordered to take a couple of Tums (calcium carbonate and sucrose) daily—this would increase calcium and therefore decrease phosphorus. More aggressive treatment for this condition would be a drug called aluminum hydroxide (Amphogel), a phosphate binder. This drug binds with phosphorus in the gut and causes it to be excreted in the stool, thereby lowering the phosphorus level. What would this do to the calcium level? You are correct! It would increase the calcium while lowering the phosphorus!

TIP: Refer to the information given for calcium.

3

OXYGENATION/
RESPIRATORY LABS

Note: Additional respiratory labs such as arterial blood gases are explained in a separate booklet titled "Interpreting Arterial Blood Gases—The Easy Way." This book is by the same author and available through Cognella.

Lactic Acid (Lactate)

Definition/Description

Lactic acid is a by-product of anaerobic metabolism. It is released when energy is needed by the cells, but there is not enough oxygen available for the normal aerobic energy cycle. The lab is used to assess for tissue oxygenation. It is also used to evaluate acidosis and to differentiate lactic acid acidosis from ketoacidosis.

It can also evaluate liver function because the liver is responsible for breaking down lactic acid. Any impairment of the liver will insult in increased lactic acid levels.

Normal Result

3–23mg/dL

Critical Abnormal Result

Greater than 31 mg/dL

Some Common Reasons for Abnormalities

Decreased:
N/A

Increased:
Cardiac failure
Diabetes
Liver impairment
Lactic acidosis
Pulmonary embolism
Shock
Strenuous exercise

Nursing Implications/Responsibilities

Client should be instructed not to eat or drink anything except water for eight to ten hours before the test. The client should be instructed not to exercise for several hours prior to the test.

4

HEMATOLOGY (OTHER THAN THE ONES THAN THE ONES DISCUSSED IN CBC)

Coagulation Studies

Prothrombin Time (PT)

Definition/Description

The prothrombin time (PT) lab is used to assess for coagulation status of the extrinsic coagulation pathway. It monitors factors II, V, VII, and X. It also is used to monitor the effectiveness of warfarin* (Coumadin) therapy.

Normal Result

10–13 seconds

Critical Abnormal Result

Greater than 27 seconds

Some Common Reasons for Abnormalities

Increased:

Liver disease
Disseminated intravascular coagulation (DIC)
Vitamin K deficiency

Warfarin therapy: Bear in mind that you should EXPECT the PT to be elevated during warfarin therapy. This is expected—you should follow the guidelines for International Normalized Ratio (INR), which follows next. PT and INR go hand in hand during warfarin therapy, and INR is the gold standard.

Also be aware than certain drugs may alter PT results. Antibiotics and acetaminophen are two common ones that can cause PT results to fluctuate.

Nursing Implications/Responsibilities

If your patient is on warfarin, review the items you will need to include for patient education. Patients will have to avoid foods rich in vitamin K such as dark green leafy vegetables. Why? Warfarin works by blocking vitamin K in the body because factors of the extrinsic clotting system need vitamin K to work effectively. You would not want to give a patient vitamin K if the warfarin is working by blocking it, thereby reducing efficiency of clotting factors. This brings us to a critical thinking question. If a patient overdoses on warfarin, what drug could we give as an antidote? You are correct again! Vitamin K!

Since patients have an increased tendency to bleed on warfarin, aspirin products should be avoided!

International Normalized Ratio (INR)

Definition/Description

This lab goes hand in hand with the prothrombin time (PT) lab. In fact, its result is derived from the PT value. It is used to monitor the effectiveness of warfarin (Coumadin) therapy.

For years, the only way to monitor the effect of warfarin was through the use of the prothrombin time. Labs used various instruments and reagents to measure this, and the results were quite varied. A method to help standardize results was needed. In the early 1980s, a committee was formed through the

World Health Organization (WHO), and this committe
algorithm that would arrive at comparable results no matte.
methods were used. The laboratory could simply refer to the in.
provided by the WHO and "standardize" its results. The formula used ν.
INR = (patient PT result/normal patient average)[ISI]. ISI in the formula stands
for international sensitivity index. Again, all of this is beyond the scope of this
basic lab book. This information gives you some idea as to what the INR is.
However, at this point, you need not dwell on how to calculate. I bet you are
saying, "Thank goodness!"

Normal Result

Less than 2 for clients not on warfarin
2–3 for clients on warfarin for venous thrombus, pulmonary embolism,
valvular heart disease, and atrial fibrillation
2.5–3.5 for clients on warfarin who have mechanical heart valves

Critical Abnormal Result

Greater than 5

Some Common Reasons for Abnormalities

Decreased:
Lack of medication compliance
Diet
Other medications

Increased:
Lack of medication compliance
Diet
Other medications

Nursing Implications/Responsibilities

Again, remember that certain drugs can cause the INR to fluctuate. Two
common ones are antibiotics and acetaminophen.

if INR is increased, bleeding precautions may need to be implemented while an adjustment in medication is made. Also, vitamin K or fresh frozen plasma may be indicated. Also bear in mind that even if INR is not increased, when a patient is on warfarin, fall prevention is VERY important. Even a minor fall can cause a bleed; internally, a cerebral bleed is possible.

Partial Thromboplastin Time, Activated (PTT or Sometimes Denoted as APTT)

Definition/Description

This lab is done to help assess clotting factors associated with the intrinsic coagulation pathway. This pathway now is known as the contact activation pathway. These clotting factors are: factors VIII, IX, XI, and XII, as well as the common pathway factors: factors I, II, V, and X. Von Willebrand factor (VIII-C) is also a part of the intrinsic coagulation pathway.

This lab is used to monitor the effectiveness of heparin, as heparin interferes with the function of some of the above factors, especially factor II.

Normal Result

25 to 35 seconds

Critical Abnormal Result

Greater than 70 seconds (unless, of course, if on heparin)

Some Common Reasons for Abnormalities

Decreased:

N/A

Heparin therapy: Usually, with heparin therapy given IV, the PTT should be 1.5–2.5 times the control (which will be listed on the lab sheet)
Hemophilia A (deficiency of factor VIII)
Hemophilia B (deficiency of factor IX)
Hemophilia C (deficiency of factor XI)
Von Willebrand's disease
Liver Problems
DIC
Hemodialysis clients (due to the effects of heparin during dialysis)

Nursing Implications/Responsibilities

The nurse must ALWAYS monitor the PTT when a client is receiving heparin. These two go together like bread and butter! Remember, with heparin therapy, the nurse should expect the PTT to be elevated 1.5–2.5 times the control, but no higher. The nurse should realize that sometimes the PTT will not be monitored for a client receiving heparin once or twice a day by the subcutaneous route. This is because the dosage is so small.

The nurse must remember that if a heparin drip is being administered and the PTT does NOT increase, this is a red flag. The client must be assessed for HIT (heparin-induced thrombocytopenia). This can be one of the first signs. The nurse immediately should notify the health-care provider who will probably order a platelet level. If platelet levels are decreasing, this is another red flag for HIT! Also, another lab that can be ordered is one checking for specific antibodies that will diagnose HIT. These antibodies are known as PF4 antibodies. If HIT is the diagnosis, the health-care provider will order the heparin to be discontinued and most likely order platelets to be administered. Another type of anticoagulant will have to be ordered until the antibodies are no longer present.

Fibrinogen

This lab test is done when some type of bleeding/clotting disorder is suspected. This lab test can assist in identifying a disorder of this type. In the final steps of the coagulation cascade, thrombin converts fibrinogen to fibrin, which is ultimately the blood clot. Without adequate fibrinogen, it would be hard for the body to make a blood clot. Fibrinogen is made in the liver.

Normal Result

200–400 mg/dL

Critical Abnormal Result

Less than 80 mg/dL

Some Common Reasons for Abnormalities

Decreased:

DIC
Liver disease
Congenital fibrinogen deficiency

Increased:

Inflammatory conditions
Cancers
Stroke
Pregnancy

Nursing Implications/Responsibilities

Since fibrinogen is increased in certain instances such as inflammatory conditions and stroke, fibrinogen can be used to assess for risk factors for vascular problems or stroke.

Bottom line: Decreased fibrinogen leads to a risk for bleeding. The nurse will need to initiate bleeding precautions. Cryoprecipitate and/or fresh frozen plasma may be ordered.

Bottom line: Increased fibrinogen increases the client's risk for clotting. Heparin may be ordered. The nurse must assess for microvascular thrombus formation. How would the nurse assess for this? Signs and symptoms would be: oliguria, tachycardia, cyanosis, loss of pulse, and signs of pulmonary embolus (shortness of breath, decreasing oxygen saturation).

Fibrin-Split Products (Sometimes Called Fibrin Degradation Products)

Definition/Description

This lab is used to assess for various conditions associated with clotting such as PE, DIC, and DVT. It also is used to check the effectiveness of fibrinolytic drugs.

Fibrin-split products also are known as fibrin degradation products. These products appear after clotting has taken place. When a clot is formed, the fibrinolytic system is activated as a check and balance to keep the clot from becoming too large and/or to prevent widespread clotting all over the body. Remember, many functions of the body have these checks and balances.

Normal Result

Less than 5 mcg/mL

Critical Abnormal Result

N/A

N/A

DIC
Renal transplant rejection
Pulmonary embolus (PE)
Deep vein thrombosis (DVT)
Postcardiac surgery
Any condition causing tissue injury

Nursing Implications/Responsibilities

The balance between coagulation and anticoagulation has been altered, so the nurse will be involved with either implementing therapies for one or both of these conditions. Bleeding precautions may be indicated if DIC is present. Therapies to promote tissue perfusion also may be indicated.

D-Dimer

Definition/Description

This lab is used to assist in diagnosing PE, DIC, DVT, and other conditions where tissue injury has occurred.

The D-dimer is a by-product of fibrin-split products. It is used to build evidence that clotting has occurred, that the fibrinolytic system has been activated, and that clots are being broken down.

The D-dimer and fibrin-split products labs actually can be used together to help diagnose certain conditions. This, again, is beyond the scope of this book.

0–0.5 mcg/mL FE

N/A

N/A

Deep vein thrombosis (DVT)
Pulmonary embolus (PE)
Disseminated intravascular coagulation (DIC)
Recent surgery
Neoplastic disease
Thrombolytic therapy

Supportive care
Bleeding precautions

Iron Studies

Iron (Serum Iron)

Essentially, this lab is ordered to differentiate between the various types of anemias, to assess blood loss, or to diagnose iron overload.

Iron in the serum is bound to a protein called transferrin. This protein transports the iron to hemoglobin, the GI tract, and to the liver or spleen for storage. The body acquires iron through ingestion of food. Only a small percentage is absorbed, and the rest is eliminated. Decreased levels of iron and increased levels of iron are both clinically significant.

Iron fundamentally is recycled—that is why only a small percentage has to be absorbed from food. Although red blood cells are destroyed after 120 days in circulation, the iron is saved and recycled. However, with blood loss, this does not happen. Anytime you have a client with blood loss, think iron loss! These two go together like bread and butter too!

Iron overload is clinically significant as well. Iron can accumulate in organs and cause damage, especially to the heart and liver. Think possible iron over-load with excessive blood transfusions. These contain iron!

Normal Result

Adult male: 65–175 mcg/dL
Adult female: 50–170 mcg/dL

Critical Abnormal Result

Mild toxicity: Greater than 350 mcg/dL
Serious toxicity: Greater than 400 mcg/dL
Lethal: Greater than 1000 mcg/dL

Some Common Reason for Abnormalities

Decreased:
Iron-deficiency anemia
Blood loss
Kidney disease
Pregnancy
Malnutrition
Cancer
Acute and chronic infections (iron is used as food for organisms)

Acute iron poisoning

Excessive blood transfusions

Lead toxicity (displaces iron and causes it to be released into serum)

Nursing Implications/Responsibilities

For the best and most accurate results for this lab, fasting is preferred—nothing by mouth after midnight before the lab is drawn in the morning.

Remember all the patient education the nurse must do when iron is given. Always think constipation! Therefore, fluids and a stool softener probably will be indicated. Iron should be given between meals if it can be tolerated, as this allows for better absorption. Also, remember that vitamin C is needed for absorption, so this vitamin may be ordered by the health-care provider. If not, the medication can be given with orange juice to supply the vitamin C.

Iron can be given IV, IM, and PO. If given IV, consult with the pharmacist for proper administration procedure, as allergic reactions can occur! If given IM, think deep IM, and use the Z track method. If given as a liquid PO, give with juice or water and through a straw, as it will stain teeth! A client will not be happy if his or her teeth are orange!

Remember to think iron overload with excessive blood transfusions. Some of the conditions where this may occur are: trauma patients, patients with thalassemia, or patients with aplastic anemia.

The treatment for iron overload may be a chelating agent—deferoxamine mesylate (Desferal). This medication binds to iron and causes it to be excreted from the body in the urine and stool. Therefore, you, as the nurse should beware! Urine and stools will be red! This demonstrates that the medication is effective!

Total Iron-Binding Capacity (TIBC)

This lab is used to help validate the presence of iron-deficiency anemia. It also is used to evaluate the effectiveness of therapy when iron is being replaced. The serum iron lab and TIBC lab have an inverse relationship.

TIP: This is an easy way to remember this:

1. Think of TIBC as a bus with lots of seats.
2. The seats are made up of transferrin, as this is the protein that carries iron in the serum.
3. When iron in the serum is low, many seats will be available, so TIBC will be high.
4. When iron in the serum is high, few seats will be available, so TIBC will be low.

Although transferrin and TIBC are NOT the same thing, you will not go wrong by thinking of them interchangeably.

Normal Result

250–350 mcg/dL

Critical Abnormal Result

N/A

Some Common Reasons for Abnormalities

Decreased:

Iron overload
Hemolytic anemias
Thalassemia

Increased:

Iron-deficiency anemia
Pregnancy

Sometimes the health-care provider will calculate the iron saturation percentage. This is done by using the value for the serum iron, dividing it by the TIBC value, and multiplying this by 100. The normal value for iron saturation is 20–50%.

Ferritin

Definition/Description

This lab is ordered to evaluate anemias, especially iron-deficiency anemia.

Ferritin is actually a protein made in the liver, spleen, and bone marrow. Stored iron is bound to ferritin. When iron is needed, ferritin releases it to transferrin, the serum carrier, and it is taken to where it is needed. The amount of ferritin in circulation is usually proportional to the amount of stored iron. Therefore, by measuring ferritin levels, the health-care provider can have an indication of the amount of stored iron that is available. Loss of stored iron indicates iron-deficiency anemia that has been occurring over a period of time or some type of storage problem.

Normal Result

This varies according to gender and age.
Adult male: 20–250 ng/mL
Adult female (age 18–39): 10–120 ng/mL
Adult female (over 40): 12–263 ng/mL

Critical Abnormal Result

N/A

Iron-deficiency anemia

Excessive menstrual periods

Hemodialysis

Frequent blood transfusions

Oral or parenteral administration of iron

Hemochromatosis

Inflammation

Liver disease

Cancer (causes ferritin inside cells to leak)

Fasting for 12 hours before this lab may be preferred. This produces more accurate results.

Sickle-Cell Labs

Sickle-Cell Screening Test

This is a lab done to assess for hemoglobin S (Hgb S). The test will be positive for those with sickle-cell anemia and for those with sickle-cell trait. Hgb S will be present in both. This condition is inherited.

Sickle-cell trait is heterozygous, which means one gene is normal (Hgb A) and the other gene is an altered hemoglobin (Hgb S). Usually, individuals with the trait have no outward signs and symptoms. However, they are carriers and can pass the Hgb S gene on to their offspring.

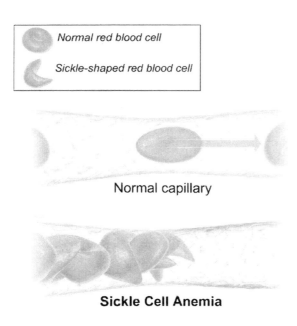

| | Normal red blood cell |
| | Sickle-shaped red blood cell |

Normal capillary

Sickle Cell Anemia

Figure 4-1 Sickle Cell Anemia

Sickle-cell anemia is homozygous recessive, which means both genes are Hgb S. Individuals have the signs and symptoms of sickle-cell anemia. "Normal" Hgb is Hgb A. Hgb S becomes "sickled" in the presence of low oxygen and will become "trapped" in blood vessels, causing great pain and circulatory problems. Can you imagine what "sickled" cells could do to the kidneys?

Sickle-cell anemia is a hemolytic anemia. The spleen identifies that the hemoglobin is structurally different and destroys it before the normal lifespan of 120 days. Clients with sickle-cell anemia have a low Hgb and Hct but adjust to it to a certain extent.

Normal Result

Negative: No Hgb S found

Critical Abnormal Result

N/A

Sickle-cell anemia

Sickle-cell trait

Nursing Implications/Responsibilities

This test also will be positive in clients with thalassemia. If this test is positive, further follow-up will be indicated with an Hgb electrophoresis. Refer to that lab information, which is included next.

Hemoglobin Electrophoresis

Definition/Description

This lab is ordered when some type of hemoglobinopathy is suspected. A hemoglobinopathy is a genetic defect in one of the structural chains of hemoglobin. The most common ones are the hemolytic anemias—sickle-cell anemia and thalassemia. This test actually identifies the various types of hemoglobin present. The types of hemoglobin are as follows: Hgb A, Hgb A_2, Hgb F, Hgb C, Hgb D, Hgb E, Hgb S, and Hgb H. Hgb A is the "normal" hemoglobin. Hgb S is found in sickle-cell anemia or sickle-cell trait. Varying amounts of Hgb A_2 are found with the beta thalassemias. Hgb H is found with the alpha thalassemias. Hgb F is a fetal hemoglobin that decreases significantly after three to four months of age but can return with such conditions as leukemia, thalassemia, and other unstable hemoglobin conditions. The remaining hemoglobins are found in other hemoglobinopathies but are more complicated and detailed than the scope of this book.

Normal Result

Hgb A > than 95%

Hgb A_2 – 1.5–3.7 %

Hgb F – < than 2%

N/A

Decreased:

N/A (except if Hgb A is decreased!)

Increased:

Hgb S: Sickle-cell trait or sickle-cell anemia (see comment below under nursing implications)

Hgb A_2: Beta thalassemias

Hgb H: Alpha thalassemias

Hgb F: Conditions such as leukemia, thalassemia, or other unstable hemoglobin conditions

Nursing Implications/Responsibilities

The test generally has to show an Hgb S content of 80–100% for a diagnosis of sickle-cell anemia.

The test generally has to show an Hgb S content of around 40% or less for a diagnosis of sickle-cell trait.

Miscellaneous Hematology Labs

Reticulocyte Count

Definition/Description

This lab usually will be done after a CBC if the red blood cell count, Hgb, and Hct are low. This lab is done to monitor activity of the bone marrow as far as making red blood cells. It also is used to monitor the effectiveness of therapy with the various anemias.

Reticulocytes are slightly immature red blood cells. They are formed in the bone marrow and released into the blood to mature. They mature in approximately two days. The bone marrow tries to "normalize" the red blood cell count by either releasing or holding onto reticulocytes. This lab is the best one for determining if therapy for anemia is working because the reticulocyte count will increase before the red blood cell count, hemoglobin, or hematocrit.

Normal Result

Percentage: 0.8–2.5%
Absolute count: 0.02–0.10 (10^6 cells/microL)

Critical Abnormal Result

N/A

Some Common Reasons for Abnormalities

Decreased:

Anemias
Bone marrow failure
Radiation therapy
Renal disease

Increased:

Blood loss
Hemolytic anemias
Therapy for anemias (that's working!)

Nursing Implications/Responsibilities

Fasting may be preferred for this lab. Check with your lab or health-care provider.

Image credit

- Fig. 4.1: Copyright © BruceBlaus (CC BY-SA 4.0) at https://commons. wikimedia.org/wiki/File%3ASickle_Cell_Anemia.png.

5 CARDIAC LABS

MI-Associated Labs

Troponin

Troponin is a protein found in skeletal and cardiac muscle. It can be divided into three subunits or types: troponin C, troponin I, and troponin T. Troponin I and troponin T are the only ones that are cardiac related. Troponin I is a more specific marker of cardiac than even troponin T. High levels of troponin I and troponin T can indicate a recent myocardial infarction (MI). Troponin I rises within two to six hours following an MI, peaks at 15–25 hours, slowly declines over 60–80 hours, and resolves after seven days. Troponin T usually rises within the first two to six hours following an MI and remains elevated for seven days. Generally, troponin I needs to be at least 1.4 ng/mL or higher for a diagnosis of MI.

Normal Result

Troponin I: less than 0.05 ng/mL
Troponin T: less than 0.2 ng/mL

N/A

MI is the number one reason. However, troponin also can be elevated with heart failure, ablation therapy, cardiac surgery, stenting, defibrillation, unstable angina pectoris, and basically any condition that causes myocardial damage.

As mentioned earlier in this book, normal ranges can differ from lab to lab. This is especially true for troponin levels. This is due to the different reagents used. Definitely refer to your lab's normal values before taking any action for troponin results!

TIP: The higher the troponin level, the greater the tissue damage.

Creatine Kinase (CK Total and CK MB)

Creatine kinase is an enzyme that exists in skeletal and cardiac muscle. Also, there are very small amounts found in the brain and lungs. CK total can be divided into three different types. These different types are termed isoenzymes. The isoenzymes are as follows: BB, which is found mainly in the brain; MM, found mainly in skeletal muscle; and MB, which is mainly found in cardiac muscle. Therefore, the MB isoenzyme is the one that is used for determining cardiac involvement. However, the total CK has to be done first in order to separate the various isoenzymes by electrophoresis. When cardiac muscle is damaged, the isoenzyme, MB, is released into the blood and is therefore elevated. Levels rise and fall in a predictable manner.

Normal Results

Males: 50–204 units/L
Females: 36–160 units/L

CK-MB
0–4% (by electrophoresis)
0–3 ng/mL (by immunoassay)
0–2.5 (CK-MB index)

Critical Abnormal Results

N/A

Some Common Reasons for Abnormalities

Decreased:
N/A

Increased:
MI
Heart failure
Myocarditis
Tachycardia

Nursing Implications/Responsibilities

With damage, CK-MB usually appears within four to six hours following the injury. It peaks 15–20 hours following the injury and usually resolves in two to three days.

Remember: when assessing for cardiac injury, the nurse must look at the CK-MB component. CK is NOT cardiac specific!

Myoglobin

This lab may be ordered where there is suspected skeletal or cardiac injury. The injury could be from ischemia, inflammation, or trauma.

Myoglobin is a protein found in skeletal and cardiac muscle. It is released after injury to skeletal or cardiac muscle. It can be measured a few hours after injury. In an MI, it rises within two to three hours after the injury, peaks in 8–12 hours, and then decreases after 24 hours. It peaks sooner than troponin but is not specific to cardiac and does not stay elevated as long.

Normal Results

Male: 28–72 ng/mL
Female: 25–58 ng/mL

Critical Abnormal Results

N/A

Some Common Reasons for Abnormalities

Decreased:

Myasthenia gravis
Rheumatoid arthritis

Increased:

MI
Rhabdomyolysis
Cardiac surgery
Burns
Exercise
IM injections
Kidney failure

A urine test for myoglobin may also be ordered.

Heart Failure Associated Labs

Brain Natriuretic Peptide (BNP)

Definition/Description

This lab is used to help diagnose heart failure.

Brain natriuretic peptide is a neurohormone that is produced in the ventricles of the heart during increased volume and increased ventricular pressure. It is an antagonist to the renin-angiotensin-aldosterone mechanism.

Normal Results

Less than 100 pg/mL

Critical Abnormal Results

N/A

Some Common Reasons for Abnormalities

Decreased:
N/A

Increased:
Heart failure
MI
Cardiac inflammation

Nesiritide (Natrecor) is a synthetic form of BNP. Therefore, BNP results must be interpreted with caution if clients are receiving or have been receiving this drug. BNP levels also may be increased above normal ranges in elderly adults.

TIP: Generally, a BNP > 800 pg/mL is needed for the health-care provider to diagnose heart failure.

Cardiovascular Risk Assessment Labs

Lipid Profile

Definition/Description

A lipid profile is a common lab test and is used to assess a client's risk of cardiovascular disease. It consists of measurement of total cholesterol and triglycerides. There are two types of cholesterol that make up total cholesterol: high-density lipoproteins (HDL) and low-density lipoproteins (LDL). Think of HDLs as being the "good" cholesterol. I remember it as being the "happy" cholesterol! Think of LDLs as the "bad cholesterol." I recall it being called the "lousy" cholesterol. Too much of it can cause plaque buildup on the walls of arteries!

Cholesterol is obtained from a client's diet but also is made in the liver and intestinal mucosa. Triglycerides mainly are composed of fatty acids, and most come from foods.

Normal Results

Total Cholesterol

Excellent: < 200 mg/dL
Borderline: 200–239 mg/dL
Bad: >240 mg/dL

Excellent: > 60 mg/dL
Acceptable: 40–60 mg/dL
Bad: <40 mg/dL

Excellent: < 100 mg/dL
Acceptable: 100–129 mg/dL
Borderline: 130–159 mg/dL
Bad: 160–189 mg/dL
Very bad: >190 mg/dL

Normal: < 150 mg/dL
Borderline: 150–199 mg/dL
Bad: 200–499 mg/dL
Very bad: > 500 mg/dL

Critical Abnormal Results

N/A

However, very low cholesterol can be as clinically significant as very high levels. Total cholesterol levels less than 120 and LDL levels less than 50 can inhibit vitamin D in the body and also cause mental health issues.

Some Common Reasons for Abnormalities (for Cholesterol and Triglycerides)

Decreased:

Malnutrition
Hyperthyroidism
End-stage liver disease

Diet high in fat and cholesterol

Cirrhosis

Metabolic syndrome

Obesity

Gout

Hypothyroidism

MI

Nursing Implications/Responsibilities

Fasting is preferred for this lab for the most accurate results. If fasting has not occurred before the lab and if the total cholesterol result is 200 mg/dL or greater, a repeat test should be performed with the client fasting after midnight.

Education is very important. Items that should be discussed include proper diet, exercise, medication compliance, and loss of weight if indicated.

Homocysteine

Definition/Description

This lab is done to assess a client's risk for cardiovascular disease, venous thrombosis, and stroke.

Homocysteine is an amino acid that is usually broken down rapidly in a process requiring vitamin B_{12} and folate. If homocysteine is not broken down correctly or if vitamin B_{12} or folate is deficient, blood vessels are damaged, increasing the risk of plaque formation. Risk for blood clots increases, and therefore the risk of stroke increases.

Normal Results

4.6–11.2 micromol/L

Critical Abnormal Results

N/A

Some Common Reasons for Abnormalities

N/A

Coronary artery disease
Folic acid deficiency
Vitamin B_{12} deficiency
Peripheral vascular disease
Cerebrovascular disease

Nursing Implications/Responsibilities

Education requiring reducing the risk of cardiac problems and stroke is needed. Items that should be discussed include diet, exercise, blood pressure control, and loss of weight if indicated.

A multivitamin containing B_{12} and folate may be ordered by the health-care provider.

Liver Labs (Other than Those Covered in CMP)

Ammonia

Definition/Description

This lab is ordered to evaluate liver function. It can be used to assess for impending hepatic encephalopathy in the presence of known liver disease. It also can be used to monitor the effectiveness of medications given to decrease ammonia levels.

Ammonia comes from the breakdown of proteins. Bacteria in the digestive tract break proteins into nitrogen compounds. Some are used to repair cells, and the rest (ammonia) is taken to the liver. The liver processes the ammonia into urea, where it is then taken to the kidneys to be eliminated from the body.

Normal Results

19–60 mcg/dL or < 50 umol/L

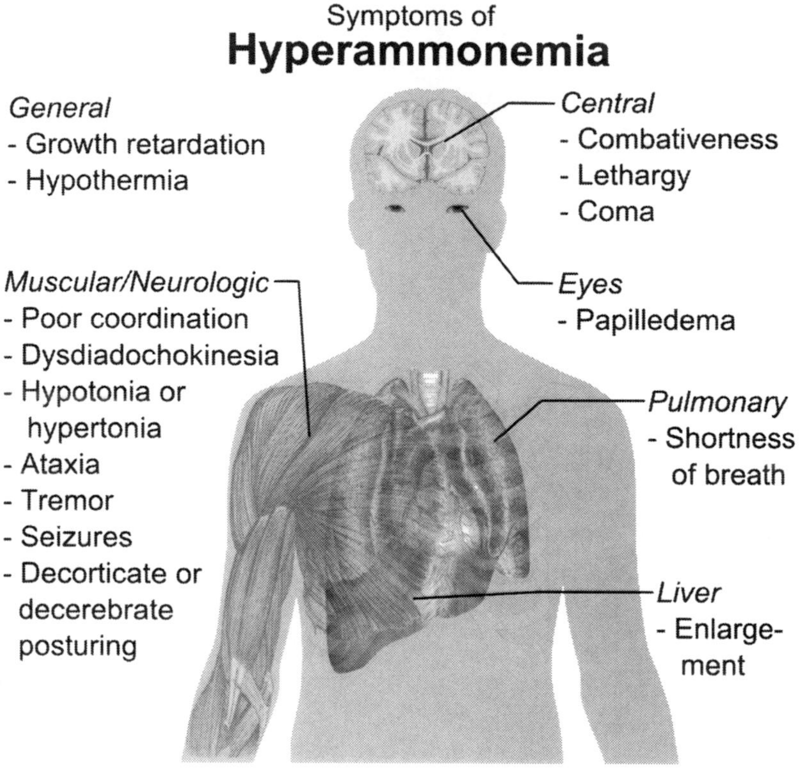

Symptoms of
Hyperammonemia

General
- Growth retardation
- Hypothermia

Central
- Combativeness
- Lethargy
- Coma

Muscular/Neurologic
- Poor coordination
- Dysdiadochokinesia
- Hypotonia or
  hypertonia
- Ataxia
- Tremor
- Seizures
- Decorticate or
  decerebrate
  posturing

Eyes
- Papilledema

Pulmonary
- Shortness
  of breath

Liver
- Enlarge-
  ment

Figure 6-1 Symptoms of Hyperammonemia

Critical Abnormal Results

Ammonia is toxic to the central nervous system and can result in encephalopathy at levels around 100 umol/L.

Some Common Reasons for Abnormalities

Decreased:
N/A

Increased:
Kidney problem
Liver problem such as cirrhosis or hepatitis
Stress

Hemolysis will show a false increased ammonia level because higher ammonia levels are found in the cells. Therefore, the specimen should be placed on ice and taken to the lab for interpretation immediately.

Remember—increased ammonia levels are toxic to the brain!

Lactalose is a major/common treatment. Be sure to review how this medication works and how the ammonia is decreased!

Hepatitis Labs

Hepatitis A Antibody

Definition/Description

This lab is ordered to diagnose present or past infection with hepatitis A. The lab will check for antibodies for hepatitis A. If the antibody is present and it is of the IgM type, this means the infection is current. If the antibody is of the IgG type, this means the client has had the infection in the past.
Hepatitis A is a hardy virus. It survives on hands and is only destroyed by high temperature or bleach. It is spread by the fecal-oral route and through contaminated food and water.

Signs and symptoms appear quickly and last about a week. Signs and symptoms can be flu-like.
A client cannot become a carrier for this type of hepatitis. Once a client has the disease, he or she has permanent immunity.

Normal Results

Negative: No detection of antibodies (anti-HAV)

Critical Abnormal Results

N/A

Positive: Antibodies present—IgM = current infection; IgG = past infection

Nursing Implications/Responsibilities

This disease usually is spread by ingestion of contaminated water and food. If exposed to acquiring hepatitis A, IgG immunoglobulins may be given to try to prevent it.

Hepatitis B Antigen and Antibody

Definition/Description

This lab is ordered to screen for present and past infection with Hepatitis B.

Hepatitis B is spread through blood-to-blood contact. Consequently, some modes of transmission are as follows: unprotected sex, needle sharing, cuts and sores (person to person), and blood products (mainly before 1992).

With this type of infection, some individuals can become chronic carriers. Almost half of the individuals infected with hepatitis B are asymptomatic. With hepatitis B, the first marker to appear in the serum is hepatitis B surface antigen (HBsAg). It usually appears within 8–12 weeks after infection. The client is infectious when this antigen is present in the serum. Liver enzymes will be elevated.

When the liver enzymes return to normal, usually this HBsAg becomes un-detectable. If it is still detectable, the client is probably going to be a chronic carrier and will be able to continue to transmit the disease. Hepatitis Be antigen (HBeAg) appears in the serum around 10–12 weeks following the infection. It is a sign of viral replication and is found in both acute and carrier states. Clients who are positive for the hepatitis Be antigen are infectious, too!

The hepatitis Be antibody (HBeAB) usually appears around 14 weeks or so after exposure. The appearance of this antibody suggests resolution of the infection and reduction in the ability to transmit the disease.

While all of the above has been happening, at around six to 14 weeks following exposure, IgM hepatitis B core antibody (HBcAb) appears. It is not an indicator of recovery or immunity. However, it does indicate past or current infection.

Hepatitis B surface antibody (HBsAb) appears after HBsAg disappears (remember, this was the very first marker to appear). The hepatitis B surface antibody does represent recovery and immunity to the virus.

Normal Results

Negative
No surface antigen, e antigen, or core antibody to hepatitis B detected

Critical Abnormal Results

N/A

Some Common Reasons for Abnormalities

Positive: HBsAg, HBeAg, or HBcAb present (hepatitis B)

Nursing Implications/Responsibilities

Universal precautions will protect the health-care provider from this disease. Health-care workers are further protected by eliminating the use of needles with clients as much as possible. Additionally, taking the hepatitis B vaccine is very important for prevention in acquiring the disease.

Hepatitis C Antibody

Definition/Description

This lab is employed to detect antibodies to hepatitis C. Usually, the enzyme-linked immunosorbent assay (ELISA) is used to check for the antibodies (anti-HCV). If positive, a confirmatory test using the recombinant immunoblot assay (RIBA) is performed.

Antibodies are usually detected in 50% of clients within four to six weeks of infection. The remaining clients test positive within one year.

Transmission for hepatitis C occurs with blood-to-blood contact. As a result, it can be spread through such methods as sexual contact or through the use of dirty needles. Health-care workers can contract through needle sticks.

A large majority of the clients with hepatitis C become carriers. These individuals have a high risk of having chronic liver disease and developing hepatic cancer.

Normal Results

Negative

No detection of antibodies for hepatitis C

Critical Abnormal Results

N/A

Some Common Reasons for Abnormalities

Positive

Antibodies detected for hepatitis C

Nursing Implications/Responsibilities

Universal precautions will protect the health-care worker against hepatitis C.

Hepatitis D Antibody

Definition/Description

This lab is ordered to detect antibodies to hepatitis D. It can detect present and past infection. If the infection is current, the antibody will be of the IgM type. If the infection has occurred in the past, the antibody will be an IgG type. Antibodies usually are present within a few days of infection.

Hepatitis D is a chronic type infection. This type of hepatitis needs hepatitis B as its helper. Therefore, it is very similar in many ways to hepatitis B.

Negative for antibodies to hepatitis D

N/A

Positive for hepatitis D antibodies indicates present or past infection with hepatitis D

Universal precautions will protect the health-care worker from hepatitis D.

Hepatitis E Antibody

This lab is ordered to diagnose hepatitis E. It looks for antibodies to the virus (anti-HEV). This type of hepatitis is rare and is sometimes called the traveler's hepatitis. It is contracted through consumption of food or water contaminated with fecal material. It is usually self-limiting and resolves within four to six weeks. It does not result in chronic infection. Symptoms include jaundice, lack of appetite, and malaise. Treatment involves supportive care, rest, and hydration.

Negative: No detection of antibodies for hepatitis E

Critical Abnormal Results

N/A

Some Common Reasons for Abnormalities

Positive for antibodies to hepatitis E indicates hepatitis E

Nursing Implications/Responsibilities

Standard precautions are all that is needed with this type of hepatitis. It is unlikely that it can be spread from person to person. It is acquired through consuming food or water contaminated with feces. If suspected exposure occurs, the person may be given IgG immunoglobulins to try to prevent the development of this type of hepatitis.

Image credit

- Fig. 6.1:https://commons.wikimedia.org/wiki/File%3ASymptoms_of_hyperammonemia.png. Copyright in the Public Domain.

7 PANCREATIC LABS

Pancreatic Enzymes Labs

Amylase

Definition/Description

Amylase is an enzyme. It is made by the salivary glands and the pancreas. Usually, it is found in the bloodstream in low amounts unless there is some type of blockage in the salivary glands or the pancreas.

Normal Result

30–110 units/L

Critical Abnormal Result

N/A

Some Common Reasons for Abnormalities

Decreased:
Hepatic disease
Pancreatectomy
Toxemia of pregnancy

Salivary gland inflammation

Pancreatitis

Pancreatic cancer

Acute appendicitis

Alcoholism

Intestinal obstruction

Biliary tract disease

Nursing Implications/Responsibilities

To determine if the problem is in the pancreas or salivary glands, review the next lab that follows.

Lipase

Definition/Description

Lipase is an enzyme, and it is ONLY made by the pancreas. It is usually ordered therefore along with amylase to help differentiate problems with the salivary glands or the pancreas (since amylase is made in the salivary glands and the pancreas). In other words, if amylase and lipase are both elevated, the problem lies in the pancreas. If amylase is elevated, but lipase is not, the problem probably lies in the salivary glands.

Normal Result

0–60 units/L

Critical Abnormal Result

N/A

Pancreatitis

Pancreatic cancer

Serum lipase is the most specific test for pancreatitis.

Glucose Labs

Fasting Glucose

This usually is the first lab that will be ordered to check for diabetes or prediabetes. It is a screening lab. It measures blood glucose level after the client has not eaten or drank anything but water for at least the previous eight hours.

Less than 126 mg/dL

Less than 40 mg/dL

Greater than 400 mg/dL

Hypoglycemia

Diabetes

Prediabetes

Stress

Steroid use

Hyperthyroidism

Nursing Implications/Responsibilities

If fasting glucose level is between 100mg/dL and 125 mg/dL and the oral glucose tolerance test (OGTT) is between 140–199 mg/dL two hours after the beginning of the test, or if Hgb A1c is 5.7–6.4%, the client most likely will be diagnosed with prediabetes.

Random Glucose

Definition/Description

This lab can be a screening lab when fasting has not occurred. Glucose levels do not vary much in healthy individuals. Glucose levels that vary indicate a problem and the need for additional tests.

Normal Results

Less than 200 mg/dL

Critical Abnormal Results

Less than 40 mg/dL

Greater than 400 mg/dL

Some Common Reasons for Abnormalities

Decreased:

Hypoglycemia

Diabetes

Prediabetes

Stress

Steroid use

Hyperthyroidism

Nursing Implications/Responsibilities

If a random screening glucose is elevated, the health-care provider will order a fasting glucose or hemoglobin A1C.

Oral Glucose Tolerance

Definition/Description

This lab is ordered to evaluate blood glucose levels to assist in the diagnosis of diabetes or prediabetes. It measures the body's ability to employ carbohydrates and initiate insulin production.

Normal Results

Two-hour normal result: < 200 mg/dL
A range within 140–199 mg/dL could indicate prediabetes

Critical Abnormal Results

Less than 40 mg/dL
Greater than 400 mg/dL

Some Common Reasons for Abnormalities

Decreased:

Hypoglycemia

Hypopituitarism

Malabsorption syndrome

Diabetes

Cushing's disease

Pancreatitis

Liver disease

Kidney disease

Nursing Implications/Responsibilities

Basic procedure:

1. Fasting for 8–12 hours prior to the test.
2. Fasting glucose drawn.
3. If result from fasting glucose is 126 mg/dL or greater, this indicates diabetes, so test will be canceled and health-care provider should be notified.
4. If the test continues, the client will drink 75 g of a glucose solution (this will be sweet and the client may become nauseated). If the client vomits, the test will be canceled.
5. The time begins when the client starts to drink the solution. The solution should be consumed in five minutes.
6. The blood glucose is drawn after two hours.

The client will need a special diet for three days before the test. A sufficient amount of carbohydrates must be consumed to prevent false results.

Client will need to be instructed not to eat, drink, exercise, or smoke for eight hours before the test.

The client may need to withhold certain medications before the test. Check specifically with the health-care provider.

This test also can be used to check for gestational diabetes during pregnancy. A different procedure is used for pregnant clients. They do not fast!

Two-Hour Postprandial Glucose

Definition/Description

This lab is not usually done to diagnose diabetes. It is done to see if a client with diabetes is taking the correct amount of insulin. However, a greater awareness of the importance of this test is emerging. The test is being recognized as one of the earliest signs of glucose metabolism abnormalities in type 2 diabetes. For diabetics, an elevated glucose result is a sign that good glycemic control is not being achieved with medications.

The two-hour postprandial glucose measures glucose levels exactly two hours after the client has started to consume a meal. Normally, blood glucose increases after one eats a meal. However, insulin is released to prevent the blood glucose level from becoming too high. Blood glucose that is too high can cause damage to eyes, kidneys, blood vessels, and nerves.

Normal Results

65–139 mg/dL
Over 140 mg/dL is abnormal

Critical Abnormal Results

Greater than 400 mg/dL

Some Common Reasons for Abnormalities

Decreased:
Hypoglycemia: Too much insulin release

Increased:
Early type 2 diabetes
Poor medication control for diabetic client

Procedure: The blood sample is drawn exactly two hours after the start of a meal. This time represents the average peak time for elevation. In nondiabetic clients, glucose can peak in 60 minutes after a meal but rarely exceeds 140 mg/dL and returns to normal levels within three hours.

C-Peptide

Definition/Description

This is a lab ordered to help distinguish between type 1 and type 2 diabetes. It does this by the assessment of beta cell function. It also can be used to evaluate the cause of hypoglycemia.

Essentially, when stimulated to release insulin, the beta cells of the pancreas convert proinsulin into two parts—insulin and C-peptide. Therefore, C-peptide correlates with insulin release and is a good indicator of how the beta cells are releasing insulin. Also, C-peptide is not affected by exogenous sources. It is excreted from the body by the kidneys.

Normal Results

0.8–3.5 ng/mL
One hour after glucose administration: 2.3–11.8 ng/mL

Critical Abnormal Results

N/A

Some Common Reasons for Abnormalities

Decreased:

Type 1 diabetes
False hypoglycemia (too much insulin being administered)

Type 2 diabetes

Renal failure (cannot excrete)

Islet cell tumor (excess insulin production)

Nursing Implications/Responsibilities

Sometimes the health-care provider may want the client to fast. At other times the health-care provider may want the lab done at certain intervals following the intake of food or glucose.

There may be dietary restrictions ordered before the test is administered.

Hemoglobin A1C (HgbA1C) (Glycated Hemoglobin)

Definition/Description

This lab is ordered to measure glycemic control over a long period of time. It measures the amount of glucose bound to hemoglobin, where it then becomes glycated hemoglobin. The higher the glucose level, the more glycated hemoglobin. Since a red blood cell lives around 120 days, the HgbA1C indicates how the blood glucose has been controlled over the past three or four months.

Normal Results

Normal: 4.0–5.5%

Prediabetes: 5.7–6.4%

Needing treatment: 6.5% or greater

Critical Abnormal Results

N/A

Some Common Reasons for Abnormalities

Decreased:

Chronic blood loss

Chronic renal failure

Hemolytic anemia

Increased:

Diabetes: poorly controlled

Cushing's disease

Medications such as steroids

Nursing Implications/Responsibilities

The ADA recommends routine testing of HgbA1C for people over age 45 who are overweight or obese. It recommends the testing of prediabetics at least yearly.

8

OTHER LABS FOR THE ENDOCRINE SYSTEM

Pituitary Labs

Adrenocorticotropic Hormone (ACTH)

Definition/Description

This lab is ordered to assess pituitary or adrenal gland dysfunctions. It also can be used to assess for ectopic ACTH-secreting tumors. A variety of different challenge tests can be employed (see below).

ACTH is released from the anterior lobe of the pituitary gland under the direction of a releasing factor from the hypothalamus. Upon its release, the adrenal cortex is stimulated to release glucocorticoids, androgens, and mineralocortocoids.

Normal Results

Male – supine position – morning specimen:
7–69 pg/mL
Female – supine position – morning specimen:
6–58 pg/mL

N/A

Decreased:

Cushing's

Exogenous steroid therapy

Increased:

Addison's disease

Congenital adrenal hyperplasia

ACTH-secreting tumor

Depression

Long-term use of corticosteroids may suppress the secretion of ACTH.

ACTH may be used in a challenge test to see if the adrenal glands are stimulated and release corticosteroids after ACTH is administered. After obtaining a baseline result for corticosteroid level, cosyntropin (a synthetic version of ACTH) is administered. If the corticosteroid level increases, this proves that the adrenal cortex is functioning and that the stimulation pathway is functioning. No increase in corticosteroid level would most likely indicate some type of pathology within the adrenal glands.

Growth Hormone

Definition/Description

This lab is ordered to evaluate the amount of growth hormone being secreted. It is used to diagnose gigantism, dwarfism, and acromegaly. Growth hormone is secreted from the anterior pituitary gland.

Adult male: 0–5 ng/mL
Adult female: 0–10 ng/mL
Male older than 60 years of age: 0–10 ng/mL
Female older than 60 years of age: 0–14 ng/mL
Keep in mind that childhood values are not discussed in this book. Abnormals within childhood would be associated with gigantism and dwarfism.

N/A

Decreased:
Dwarfism
Hypopituitarism
Adrenocortical hyperfunction (inhibits growth hormone)

Increased:
Gigantism
Acromegaly
Diabetes
Ectopic GH-secreting tumors
Hyperpituitarism

Remember to educate clients about the importance of growth charts for children. Also remember that excess growth hormone stimulates blood glucose. Consequently, excess growth hormone could be a reason for elevated glucose levels—it doesn't always have to be diabetes!

Prolactin

This is a lab ordered to try to identify the presence of a prolactin-secreting tumor. It also is ordered to try to determine the cause of lactation problems in a postpartum client.

Prolactin is secreted by the anterior lobe of the pituitary gland. It usually is elevated in pregnant or lactating females. The function of prolactin is milk production. Tumors can develop that secrete prolactin, and milk production occurs in nonpregnant individuals. Infertility is a problem also in both males and females who have this type of tumor.

Normal Results

Adult females: 4–30 ng/mL
Adult males: 4–23 ng/mL
Pregnant females: 5.3–215.3 ng/mL
Postmenopausal females: 2.424 ng/mL

Critical Abnormal Results

N/A

Some Common Reasons for Abnormalities

Decreased:
Pituitary malfunction
Sheehan's syndrome

Increased:
Ectopic prolactin-secreting tumors (lungs, kidneys)
Pituitary tumors
Amenorrhea (pathology unknown)
Anorexia nervosa (pathology unknown)
Breastfeeding
Stress

Many medications can cause increased prolactin levels, especially psychiatric medications. Refer to your main lab book for a listing of all medications.

Osmolality (Serum)

This lab is ordered to evaluate hydration and to assess acid/base balance. It is used to help diagnose metabolic, renal, and endocrine disorders. Some examples of these disorders where this lab is useful are antidiuretic hormone disorders, diabetes, and various toxic conditions.

This can be an actual measured lab or a calculated lab. The formula for the calculated one is as follows: $(2 \times NA^+) + (glucose/18) + BUN/2.8$. This lab measures the number of particles in serum. The major particles that contribute to osmolity are sodium, chloride, bicarbonate, urea, and glucose.

275–295 mOsm/kg

Less than 265 mOsm/kg
Greater than 320 mOsm/kg

Hyponatremia
Syndrome of inappropriate antidiuretic hormone (SIADH)
Water intoxication

Azotemia

Dehydration

Diabetes insipidus

Diabetic ketoacidosis

Hypernatremia

Nursing Implications/Responsibilities

The actual measured serum osmolality is normally greater than the estimated measurement. If an actual measured result is available, the health-care provider can compare its result to the estimated result. The osmolality gap is the difference between the two and is usually 5–10 mOsm/kg. If the difference is greater than 15 mOsm/kg, the health-care provider should consider toxicity by ethanol (drinking alcohol), ethylene glycol (antifreeze), or methanol (wood or nondrinking alcohol found in such things as copy machine fluids, paint thinner, octane boosters, and windshield wiper fluid).

Adrenal Labs

Aldosterone Levels

Definition/Description

This lab may be ordered to evaluate hypertension, especially in clients presenting with low potassium levels who are not on diuretics. A health-care provider, in doing this, might be suspicious of an aldosterone-secreting tumor. The renin-angiotensin pathway would be evaluated. It also may be ordered to validate aldosterone levels in clients presenting with certain signs and symptoms such as those that occur with Addison's disease.

Normal Results

Supine: 3–16 ng/dL

Upright: 7–30 ng/dL

N/A

Some Common Reasons for Abnormalities

Decreased:
Addison's disease

Increased:
Primary aldosteronism
Cushing's disease

Nursing Implications/Responsibilities

Levels generally decline as a client ages.

Sodium intake, medications, and activity could influence the outcome of this lab.

Cortisol Levels

Definition/Description

This lab is ordered to determine adrenal function. It is used to determine either a suspected excess or deficiency in cortisol such as in Cushing's disease or Addison's disease. It also is ordered to establish a baseline to be used with all the various challenge tests to determine if pathways and feedback mechanisms are functional.

Cortisol is the main glucocorticoid secreted by the adrenal cortex when ACTH is released. The highest levels occur in the morning, with the lowest levels occurring later in the day. Cortisol and ACTH are usually evaluated together, as concentrations of one can affect the other.

8 a.m. normal result: 5–25 mcg/dL
4 p.m. normal result: 3–16 mcg/dL

N/A

Addison's disease
Hypopituitarism

Cushing's disease
Adrenal adenoma
Excess ACTH production
Stress

Remember that increased cortisol levels can be one of the reasons that a client presents with hyperglycemia.

Dexamethasone Suppression Test

This is a lab ordered to check the stimulation/feedback system between the adrenal cortex and the anterior lobe of the pituitary gland. It is ordered when the health-care provider suspects some type of secreting tumor, either pituitary, adrenal, or ectopic. Refer to the information listed with cortisol in this booklet.

Less than 1.8 mcg/dL on the morning following the administration of dexamethasone (Decadron).

N/A

Ectopic source of cortisol

Procedure:

1. Get a baseline cortisol level at 8 a.m.
2. Give an oral dose of 1 mg dexamethasone (Decadron) at 11 p.m.
3. Check cortisol level on the next morning at 8 a.m.
4. Compare to the baseline cortisol level. The second level should be significantly decreased because with the excess cortisol (dexamethasone), the feedback loop would stop the secretion of ACTH from the anterior pituitary, which would stop the stimulus for the adrenal cortex to release cortisol.

Note: Clients with psychiatric illnesses may have abnormal results.

Renin Levels

Renin is secreted by the kidneys in response to low blood pressure or low sodium (Na). Renin stimulates the renin-angiotensin system and signals the adrenal cortex to secrete mineralocortocoid salt (Na). This corrects sodium deficits and increases blood pressure (because water follows the

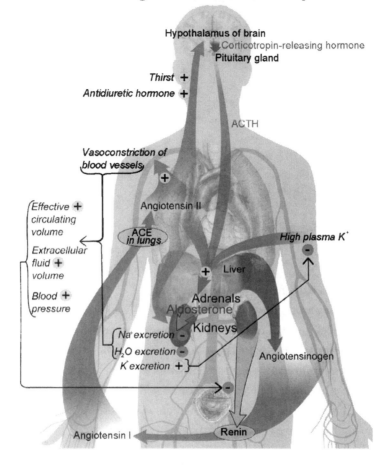

Renin-angiotensin-aldosterone system

Hypothalamus of brain

Corticotropin-releasing hormone

Pituitary gland

Thirst +

Antidiuretic hormone +

ACTH

Vasoconstriction of blood vessels

+

Angiotensin II

Effective + circulating volume

ACE in lungs

High plasma K⁺

Extracellular fluid + volume

+ Liver

Blood + pressure

Adrenals
Aldosterone

Kidneys

Na⁺ excretion −

H₂O excretion −

Angiotensinogen

K⁺ excretion +

−

Angiotensin I

Renin

Figure 8-1 Renin-angiotensin system in man shadow

sodium and increases blood pressure by increasing volume). This lab test is used most often for trying to help determine the cause of a client's hypertension.

Normal Results

Adult: 0.2–2.3ng/mL/hr.
Older adult: 1.3–4ng/mL/hr.

N/A

Cushing's disease
Aldosterone-secreting tumor

Addison's disease
Any condition where sodium is decreased or diluted (cirrhosis, heart failure, and hypotension)

Recall the normal renin pathway. Low sodium or low blood pressure causes renin release from the kidney; renin stimulates release of angiotensin I. This stimulates the release of angiotensin II. This, in turn, causes the release of aldosterone from the adrenal cortex with an end result of Na^+ and water retention. This raises the blood pressure and corrects the low sodium, and the cycle stops. Remember that an ACE inhibitor works to stop this process! An ACE inhibitor is an angiotensin-converting enzyme inhibitor! Therefore, this medication will stop sodium and water retention. Angiotensin contributes to vasoconstriction so this will be stopped too.

Catecholamines

This lab may be ordered when hypertension is present and has not responded to standard treatment. It is ordered to help diagnose a pheochromocytoma.

A pheochromocytoma is a catecholamine-secreting tumor that secretes epinephrine, norepinephrine, and dopamine, causing vasoconstriction with resulting hypertension. A pheochromocytoma is a tumor, usually benign, located on or around the adrenal medulla. The adrenal medulla normally releases catecholamines, in conjunction with the sympathetic nervous system causing the fight-or-flight response.

A pheochyromocytoma secretes catecholamines outside the normal pathways.

Normal Results

Epinephrine
Adult supine (for 30 minutes): 0–110 pg/mL
Adult standing (for 30 minutes): 0–140 pg/mL

Norepinephrine
Adult, supine (for 30 minutes): 70–750 pg/mL
Adult, standing (for 30 minutes: 200–1700 pg/mL

Dopamine
Adult, standing or supine: 0–48 pg/mL

Critical Abnormal Results

N/A

Some Common Reasons for Abnormalities

Decreased:
Parkinson's disease
Autonomic nervous system dysfunction

Increased:
Pheochromocytoma
Strenuous exercise
Neuroblastoma
Long-term bipolar disorder
Ganglioblastoma
Ganglioneuroma

Nursing Implications/Responsibilities

Catecholamines in the blood can be affected by many variables such as stress, smoking, diet, and temperature. Thus, a 24-hour urine test is more reliable. See VMA under the urine section in this booklet.

Note: If catecholamines are elevated without hypertension, the health-care provider should suspect neuroblastoma.

Thyroid Labs

Triiodothyronine (T$_3$)

Definition/Description

This lab usually is ordered if TSH is abnormal and is ordered in conjunction with T$_4$. It is ordered to help diagnose thyroid problems. The lab can measure total T$_3$, free T$_3$, or both. T$_3$ is released from the thyroid gland in smaller quantities than T$_4$. Most of it is actually formed from T$_4$. One-third of T$_4$ is converted to T$_3$ in the tissues. Like T$_4$, most of T$_3$ is bound to thyroxine-binding globulin, prealbumin, and albumin. T$_3$ is four to five times more potent than T$_4$. Both are responsible for maintaining the client in a normal thyroid state.

Normal Results

Total – Adult: 70–204 ng/dL
Total – Older adult: 40–181 ng/dL
Free – Adult – all ages: 2.6–4.8 pg/mL

Critical Abnormal Results

N/A

Hypothyroidism

Malnutrition (decreased transport proteins)

Acute disease not related to thyroid (pathology unclear)

Hyperthyroidism

T_3 toxicosis

Many medications can interfere with the results of this lab, so refer to your detailed lab book.

Thyroxine (T_4)

This lab may be ordered along with a T_3 if the TSH value is abnormal. This is used to help identify the source of thyroid problems and is used also to evaluate the effectiveness of thyroid medications.

As such, this lab can be ordered as a total T_4 or a free T_4. (See the explanation in the next paragraph.)

Thyroxine is released from the thyroid gland under the direction of TSH from the pituitary gland. Most of it is bound to prealbumin, albumin, and thyroxine-binding globulin. The remainder is free and circulates and is the "active" thyroid (less than 1%). The level of free thyroxine is proportional to the level of total thyroid. Free is considered to be the most accurate, since it is not affected by levels of globulin and albumin.

Total: 4.6–12 mcg/dL
Free: 0.8–1.5 ng/dL

For the total thyroid: less than 2 mcg/dL
For the total thyroid: greater than 20 mcg/dL

Decreased:
Hypothyroidism
Panhypopituitarism

Increased:
Hyperthyroidism
Hypothyroidism being treated with thyroid medication
Acute psychiatric illness (pathology unknown)

Remember that since the total T_4 is associated with protein, as this is the mode of transportation for most of it, the health-care provider should rely on free T_4 results if protein levels are altered.

Thyroid-Stimulating Hormone (TSH)

Definition/Description

This lab is one of the first labs ordered to assess thyroid function. Many times, it is done alone as a screening lab to see if there could be thyroid problems. It may be done along with T_4 to diagnose hypothyroidism or hyperthyroidism.

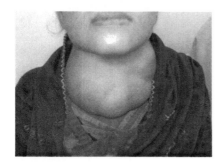

Figure 8-2 Goiter

Recall the feedback control between the pituitary gland and the thyroid gland. TSH is released from the pituitary gland if the thyroid hormone level is low. Neuroregulators will stimulate the pituitary gland to release this TSH. The TSH goes to the thyroid gland to stimulate the release of thyroid hormone. Once the thyroid level is no longer low, the neuroregulators recognize this and stop the process. If thyroid hormone is high, the neuroregulators will identify this and notify the pituitary gland to stop the release of TSH.

As a result, if the "normal" control and feedback system are working correctly, if the thyroid level is high, TSH will be decreased; if the thyroid level is low, TSH will be increased.

Normal Results

0.4–4.2 micro international units/mL

Critical Abnormal Results

N/A

Some Common Reasons for Abnormalities

Decreased:

Hyperthyroidism
Pituitary problem (TSH cannot be released; blocked)
Excessive thyroid hormone replacement

Increased:

Hypothyroidism
Ectopic TSH-producing tumor

Many medications can alter TSH levels. Some of these are amiodarone, lithium, morphine, and valproic acid. Refer to the detailed lab book for a complete listing of medications that can alter results.

Thyroid Radioactive Iodine Uptake Test

Definition/Description

This is a nuclear medicine test. It is ordered to evaluate the ability of the thyroid to concentrate iodine and make thyroid hormone. This information is used to help validate a diagnosis of hyperthyroidism or hypothyroidism.

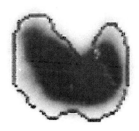

Figure 8-3 Gamma Camera Thyroid Scan

A small dose of radioactive iodine is given to the client, and scans are performed at specified intervals. Excess iodine is excreted in the urine.

Normal Results

Iodine Uptake:

2-hour absorption: 1–13%
6-hour absorption: 2–25%
24-hour absorption: 15–45%

Critical Abnormal Results

N/A

Some Common Reasons for Abnormalities

Decreased:

Hypothyroidism

Increased:
Hyperthyroidism

Nursing Implications/Responsibilities

This test is contraindicated in pregnant clients.

Recent tests containing iodine, medications containing iodine, or a diet with iodine-rich foods can alter the results of this test.

Parathyroid Gland Labs

Parathyroid Hormone

Definition/Description

This lab is ordered to validate the amount of parathyroid hormone. It can be ordered to assess damage from inadvertent removal of the parathyroid glands during thyroid or neck surgery. It also can be ordered to differentiate between parathyroid and non-parathyroid causes of hypercalcemia.

This lab can be ordered to validate suspected secondary hyperparathyroidism in chronic renal failure. Remember the pathology with this. Renal failure results in increased phosphorus because it cannot be excreted. An increase in the amount of phosphorus results in decreased calcium levels in the blood because of the inverse relationship between phosphorus and calcium. A decreased calcium level stimulates the release of parathyroid hormone, and this cycle continues.

Keep in mind that parathyroid hormone is secreted by the parathyroid glands in response to low serum calcium levels. Parathyroid hormone raises serum calcium levels by pulling calcium from the bones, causing the kidneys to hold onto and reabsorb calcium, and causing the intestines to absorb more calcium.

10–65 pg/mL

N/A

Some Common Reasons for Abnormalities

Decreased:

Hypoparathyroidism due to surgery
Autoimmune destruction of parathyroid glands
Hyperthyroidism (increases the loss of calcium from bone)
Hypomagnesium (magnesium is a calcium-channel blocker; low levels allow calcium to increase)

Increased:

Renal failure
Any condition that causes decreased serum calcium

Nursing Implications/Responsibilities

Parathyroid hormone always should be measured with calcium for proper interpretation. Vitamin D is needed for the production of parathyroid hormone.

Vitamin D

Definition/Description

This lab is ordered to assess for vitamin D deficiency or toxicity. It also is ordered to help establish the cause of any calcium or phosphorus abnormalities as well as any bone disorders.

There are two active forms of vitamin D in the body. One is vitamin D 25-dihydroxy, which comes mainly from sunlight, and is the major circulating type of vitamin D. The second type is vitamin D 1,25-dihydroxy, and it comes primarily from food where plants have absorbed the sunlight. It also occurs naturally in some foods such as fish, and some of the food supply has now been fortified with this vitamin D. It is a more active form of vitamin D, and its role is to assist parathyroid hormone and calcitonin, a hormone of the thyroid gland.

Research continues about the links between vitamin D and such diseases as multiple sclerosis, type 2 diabetes, stroke, hypertension, depression, and heart failure. Measurement of vitamin D 25-dihydroxy has been found to be a more reliable measurement of vitamin D concentrations in the blood than measurement of vitamin D 1,25-dihydroxy.

Normal Result

Vitamin D 25-dihydroxy

Deficient: Less than 20 mg/mL
Low: 20–30 ng/mL
Good: Greater than 30 ng/mL
Possible Toxic Level: Greater than 150 ng/mL

Vitamin D 1,25-dihydroxy

Good: 15–60 pg/mL

Critical Abnormal Result

For vitamin D 25-dihydroxy, a value greater than 150 ng/mL can indicate toxicity

Some Common Reasons for Abnormalities

Decreased:

Rickets
Pancreatic insufficiency

Malabsorption
Celiac disease
Bowel resection

Over-supplementation

Nursing Implications/Responsibilities

The nurse should remember that vitamin D is a fat-soluble vitamin, which means that excess is not easily removed from the body as with water-soluble vitamins. Toxicity can occur with fat-soluble vitamins and can be as significant as having deficient amounts.

Image credits

- Fig. 8.1: https://commons.wikimedia.org/wiki/File%3ARenin-angiotensin_system_in_man_shadow.svg. Copyright in the Public Domain.
- Fig. 8.2: https://commons.wikimedia.org/wiki/File%3AGoitre.jpg. Copyright in the Public Domain.
- Fig. 8.3: https://commons.wikimedia.org/wiki/File%3AGamma_Camera_Thyroid_Scan.jpg. Copyright in the Public Domain.

9 IMMUNE SYSTEM LABS

Antigen/Antibody Labs

Coombs' Antiglobulin

Definition/Description

This lab is ordered when hemolysis of red blood cells is suspected. It can be conducted using either a direct method or an indirect method.

The direct method looks for actual hemolysis of the red blood cells. This happens because of sensitization of red blood cells because of certain conditions, diseases, or drugs. The result is actual hemolysis of the red blood cell due to IgG (an immunoglobulin/antibody) or complement. This can occur in autoimmune hemolytic anemia, hemolytic disease of the newborn, from the administration of certain drugs, or infusion of the wrong type of blood. Positive results are graded 1+ to 4+, with 4+ having the most agglutination.

The indirect method identifies the presence of the antibodies causing hemolysis or the presence of complement molecules. The indirect method is used to detect maternal antibodies that could be harmful to the fetus. It also is used to determine antibody titers in Rh-negative women who have been exposed (sensitized) to Rh-positive blood. Another use of this lab using the indirect method is to check for antibodies prior to a blood transfusion.

Normal Result

Direct Method
Negative result—No positive finds of agglutination

Indirect Method
Negative result: No positive finds of agglutination or detection of unexpected antibodies of complement molecules

Critical Abnormal Result

N/A

Some Common Reasons for Abnormalities

Decreased:
N/A

Increased:
Autoimmune hemolytic anemia
Drug-induced hemolytic anemia
Hemolytic disease of the newborn
Incompatible cross match
Lymphomas
Infectious mononucleosis

Nursing Implications/Responsibilities

A hemolytic reaction—whether immune mediated or drug induced—can occur very quickly and be life threatening!

Enzyme-Linked Immunosorbent Assay (ELISA)

Definition/Description

This is the first test that the health-care provider will order to screen for human immunodeficiency virus (HIV). It detects HIV antibodies in the blood. If there is a positive result for the ELISA, the health-care provider will order a western blot test to confirm the diagnosis.

Normal Result

Negative
No detection of HIV antibodies

Critical Abnormal Result

N/A

Some Common Reasons for Abnormalities

Possible HIV infection: will need to confirm with western blot

Nursing Implications/Responsibilities

If it is confirmed that client is positive for HIV, patient education and counseling will be necessary. Client should be referred to a support group. This will be a life-changing event for the client!

Western Blot

Definition/Description

This test is used to confirm HIV after a positive ELISA test. The test is more complicated than the ELISA and more sensitive. It separates the HIV sample into individual proteins by the use of an electrical current. The separated proteins are placed on a blotting paper where specific kinds of antibodies can be detected.

Normal Result

Negative

No HIV antibodies identified

Critical Abnormal Result

N/A

Some Common Reasons for Abnormalities

If western blot is positive, client is infected with HIV.

Nursing Implications/Responsibilities

The client must be counseled and referred to a support group. HIV infection is a life-changing event!

Radioallergosorbent Test (RAST)

Definition/Description

This lab is ordered for clients with allergic reactions to try to identify the allergens responsible for the reactions. It is an alternative to skin testing, which can be painful and potentially dangerous for some clients (producing anaphylaxis).

A specific IgE immunoglobulin (antibody-like) is formed in response to an allergic reaction. This lab detects and measures certain IgE immunoglobulins specific to common allergens such as medications, animal dander, foods, dust, trees, grasses, insects, venom, mites, molds, and weeds.

Allergy absent or undetectable: Less than 0.35 kU/L
Low allergy: 0.35–0.7 kU/L
Moderate allergy: 0.71–3.5 kU/L
High allergy: 3.51–17.5 kU/L
Very high allergy: 17.5 kU/L or greater

Critical Abnormal Result

N/A

Some Common Reasons for Abnormalities

Decreased:

Asthma (endogenous)
Radiation therapy

Increased:

Allergic rhinitis
Asthma (exogenous)
Anaphylaxis
Atopic dermatitis
Eczema
Hay fever
Latex allergy

Nursing Implications/Responsibilities

If a client has had radiation therapy or a radioactive scan within the week, the test needs to be postponed for a few days, if possible. This will interfere with the test, and results likely will not be accurate.

Inflammatory Response Associated Labs

C-Reactive Protein (CRP)

This lab is ordered when an inflammatory process is suspected. It also can be ordered to help differentiate between certain disease processes, where one is inflammatory and the other is not. This lab also can be used to identify individuals at risk for coronary artery disease or peripheral vascular disease, as inflammation plays a major role with these two conditions.

CRP is nonspecific. It only demonstrates that inflammation is present; it does not diagnose.

CRP is released from the liver in the presence of inflammation. It is very sensitive and is a rapid indicator of inflammation. It also disappears very quickly when inflammation has subsided.

Less than 1 mg/dL

1–3 mg/dL

Greater than 10 mg/dL (after repeat testing)

N/A

N/A

Crohn's disease
Inflammatory bowel disease
Myocardial infarction
Rheumatoid arthritis
Systemic lupus erythematosus (SLE)
Acute bacterial infection

The health-care provider often orders this lab along with the erythrocyte sedimentation rate (ESR). However, CRP is more sensitive and rapid acting than ESR.

Procalcitonin

This is a lab ordered to assist in diagnosing a bacterial infection and to assess the risk for developing sepsis.

Procalcitonin is the precursor of the hormone, calcitonin, made by the thyroid gland. With systemic inflammatory response (SIRS), a variety of agents trigger the production of procalcitonin by non-thyroid tissues. This increase in procalcitonin is detectable within two to four hours of the development of SIRS and peaks within 12–14 hours.

Less than 0.1 ng/mL

See below under Nursing Implications/Responsibilities

Some Common Reasons for Abnormalities

Decreased:

N/A

Increased:

Septicemia

Multiorgan failure

Procalcitonin-secreting tumor

Conditions causing widespread inflammatory response such as burns or recent surgery

Nursing Implications/Responsibilities

See below for the guidelines used by the health-care provider:

Less than 0.1 ng/mL: Bacterial infection not likely present.

Less than 0.5 ng/mL: Bacterial infection possible—low risk of sepsis developing.

0.5–2ng/mL: Bacterial infection probably present—sepsis possible.

2.1–9.9 ng/mL: Bacterial infection very likely—high risk for sepsis.

10 ng/mL or greater: Bacterial infection severe—septic shock most likely.

Erythrocyte Sedimentation Rate (ESR)

Definition/Description

This lab is ordered to assist in diagnosing acute or chronic infection and acute inflammation. It is nonspecific but is often an early indicator of inflammation with a disease process. It also can be used to monitor the course of a disease and its response to therapy. ESR will decrease with improvement of disease and decreasing inflammation.

This lab works by measuring how fast red blood cells settle to the bottom of a test tube over a period of time. Little settling occurs in normal blood. However, with inflammation, it is felt that fibrinogen and other substances cause red blood cells to become heavy and sticky and to therefore settle more rapidly to the bottom of the test tube.

Normal Result

Results differ according to age and gender.

Age	Male	Female
Less than 50 years of age	0–15 mm/hr	0–25 mm/hr
50 years of age and older	0–20 mm/hr	0–30 mm/hr

Critical Abnormal Result

N/A

Some Common Reasons for Abnormalities

Decreased:
Conditions with high Hgb and red blood cell count (no space to fall and settle)

Increased:
Inflammatory diseases
Acute myocardial infarction
Systemic lupus erythematosus (SLE)
Crohn's disease
Lymphoma
Multiple myeloma
Nephritis
Rheumatoid arthritis

Nursing Implications/Responsibilities

This lab is ordered usually in conjunction with C-reactive protein. There is usually a prolonged elevation of ESR with malignancies.

Renal Blood Labs

BUN/Creatinine Ratio

Definition/Description

This is not really a lab but is a ratio calculated from the blood urea nitrogen (BUN) lab and the serum creatinine lab.

BUN reflects the balance between the amount of protein intake and the amount of protein excreted by the kidneys. BUN and serum creatinine are usually evaluated together because both normally are in fairly constant amounts and both are excreted by the kidneys. Therefore, BUN and creatinine go together like bread and butter. However, an increased BUN does not always mean kidney dysfunction. You must look at the BUN/creatinine ratio! If both BUN and creatinine are increased, the ratio will most likely be normal (within the 15:1–24:1 ratio), and this most likely indicates some type of kidney dysfunction. If only the BUN is increased, the ratio will be increased, and this indicates a non-kidney problem is causing the increase in the BUN.

The BUN/creatinine ratio is determined by dividing the BUN result by the creatinine result. The answer is the number other than 1 that you are looking for in the ratio; normal should be between 15 and 24.

Wow! This is getting difficult and confusing, so let's look at two examples!

Example #1
BUN: 55 mg/dL
Creatinine: 2.3 mg/dL
Ratio is calculated by: 55/2.3 = 23.9
The 23.9 is between the normal value of 15 and 24, so the ratio is normal. However, both the creatinine and the BUN are increased, so the conclusion is that this is probably a kidney dysfunction.

Example #2
BUN: 55 mg/dL
Creatinine: 0.8 mg/dL
Ratio is calculated by: 55/0.8 = 68.75
The 68.75 is NOT between the normal ratio of 15 and 24. The BUN is the only result that is elevated; the creatinine is within normal limits. The conclusion is that the elevation of the BUN is due to a non-kidney reason.

Normal Result

Ratio of 15:1–24:1
However, you must still look at the individual lab values—both may be abnormal as far as the normal values for BUN and creatinine. Remember here that we only are looking at the RATIO, which helps us to rule out and identify certain conditions.

Critical Abnormal Result

N/A

Some Common Reasons for Abnormalities

Ratio may be abnormal because only the BUN is decreased. Some reasons for this are:

Low-protein diet
Malnutrition
Liver failure

Ratio may be abnormal because only the BUN is increased. Some reasons for this are:
High-protein diet
Gastrointestinal bleeding
Burns

Nursing Implications/Responsibilities

The BUN/creatinine ratio also is useful in differentiating chronic renal failure from acute renal failure. In most cases of chronic renal failure, the BUN/creatinine ratio remains consistently normal.
Do not eat a lot of meat or other protein before having a lab for BUN.

Cystatin C (Cystatin 3) (CST3)

Definition/Description

This lab is ordered to assess kidney function. It can be used along with serum creatinine and the glomerular filtration rate (GFR) to get a complete picture of renal function. Additionally, this lab is used to monitor the functioning of a transplanted kidney.

This lab has just recently emerged on the scene as being useful in evaluating kidney function. It is a proteinase inhibitor that is produced by all nucleated cells in the body. It is excreted by the kidneys and does not reenter circulation. Therefore, the serum concentration of cystatin C is directly related to kidney function. It is thought by some to be a better indicator of kidney function than creatinine since its levels are not affected by age, sex, weight, and muscle mass. However, its use is not as widespread as the serum creatinine and GFR for predicting renal function.

Up to age 50: 0.56–0.9 mg/L
50 years of age and older: 0.58–1.08 mg/L

Critical Abnormal Result

N/A

Some Common Reasons for Abnormalities

Decreased:
N/A

Increased:
Decreased renal function

Nursing Implications/Responsibilities

Recently, cystatin C has been studied regarding its role in predicting the status of cardiac disease.

Glomerular Filtration Rate (GFR)

Definition/Description

The GFR is ordered to assess renal function. It actually is an estimated value based on the results of a serum creatinine lab and using other variables such as age, gender, body size, and race (African American versus non–African American).

The GFR (sometimes referred to an eGFR, since it is estimated) usually is calculated each time a serum creatinine level is ordered.

Age, gender, body size, and race are factors because the amount of creatinine is affected by muscle mass. Muscle mass decreases as a person ages. Males and many African Americans have more muscle mass generally. Also, chronic kidney disease is more prevalent in the African American population, so this has to be considered.

The only way to get an actual GFR is through a urine creatinine clearance test. This involves the collection of a 24-hour urine, which is difficult. All urine must be collected within the 24 hours, or errors will exist with the result.

Normal Result

Adult male: 85–125 mL/min/1.73m^2
Adult female: 75–115 mL/min/1.73m^2
Over 40 years of age: Decrease of 6–7 mL/min/1.73^2 each decade of life

Critical Abnormal Result

Degree of Decreased Filtration:
Borderline: 62.5–80 mL/min/1.73m^2
Slight: 52–62.5 mL/min/1.73m^2
Mild: 42–52 mL/min/1.73m^2
Moderate: 28–42 mL/min/1.73^2
Marked: Less than 28 mL/min/1.73^2

Some Common Reasons for Abnormalities

Decreased:
Chronic kidney disease
Diabetic nephropathy

Nursing Implications/Responsibilities

The nurse must monitor fluid and electrolyte balance. Additionally, the nurse must provide emotional support and refer the client to a support group.

The nurse must be involved with educating the client regarding the pathophysiology of renal failure, prevention of complications, and compliance with medications and diet.

11 URINE LABS

Renal Urine Labs

Microalbumin

Definition/Description

This is a urine lab that is used to detect early diabetes or to screen clients with diabetes or prediabetes for the development of diabetic nephropathy.

Microalbumin is albumin found in urine that is undetectable by dipstick and traditional methods. Microalbumin in urine precedes the development of nephropathy by five to seven years. Other renal tests do not detect problems this far in advance.

This lab can be done using a random urine sample or by using a 24-hour urine collection.

Normal Result

Random: Less than 30 mcg/albumin/mg creatinine

Normal: Less than 30 mg/g creatinine/24 hr

Microalbuminuria: 30–299 mg/g creatinine/24 hr

Clinical albuminuria: 300 mg or greater/g creatinine/24 hr

Critical Abnormal Result

N/A

Some Common Reasons for Abnormalities

Decreased:

N/A

Increased:

Diabetic nephropathy

Pre-eclampsia

Renal disease

Urinary tract infection

Exercise

Nursing Implications/Responsibilities

Usually, a random sample is ordered first. If the result is abnormal or suspicious, a 24-hour urine collection may be ordered. Several labs over a three-to-six month period may be ordered to confirm results, as many factors such as hydration, infection, and hyperglycemia can interfere.

The client and family will need to be educated on how to collect a 24-hour urine specimen.

Miscellaneous Urine Labs

Bence Jones Proteins

This lab usually is ordered when there are signs and symptoms of multiple myeloma or other malignant lymphomas.

With multiple myeloma, one type of white blood cell—the lymphocyte, specifically the B lymphocyte—makes one kind of IgG in excess. IgG is a type of antibody. Bence Jones proteins are a breakdown product of this type of IgG. They are filtered in the kidneys and appear in the urine. There should be NO Bence Jones proteins in the urine. If these proteins do appear, this is a sign of a diagnosis of multiple myeloma.

Bence Jones proteins are named for Henry Bence Jones, who named them in 1847.

Normal Result

No Bence Jones proteins in the urine

Critical Abnormal Result

N/A: Just report the presence of any Bence Jones proteins in the urine to the health-care provider

Some Common Reasons for Abnormalities

Presence of Bence Jones proteins in the urine: multiple myeloma

Nursing Implications/Responsibilities

Procedure:
Obtain clean-catch urine.
Collect at least 2 ounces of urine.

Schilling Test

Definition/Description

This urine and nuclear medicine lab is used to diagnose pernicious anemia. With this type of anemia, the client lacks the intrinsic factor secreted by the cells found in the lining of the stomach. The intrinsic factor is needed for vitamin B12 to be absorbed in the digestive tract. Red blood cells need B12. Without it, the red blood cells will be decreased, and the client will be anemic. However, there are other ways the client can be deficient in vitamin B12 other than lacking the intrinsic factor. The client can have other absorption problems or can be consuming a diet deficient in vitamin B12. This lab is used to differentiate the lack of the intrinsic factor from other causes.

Normal Result

"Tagged" B12 found in Step 1 (see procedure below); therefore, no lack of the intrinsic factor found

Critical Abnormal Result

N/A

Some Common Reasons for Abnormalities

"Tagged" B12 found in Step 1: anemia caused by another reason other than lack of the intrinsic factor
"Tagged" B12 not found in Step 1 but found in Step 2: anemia caused by lack of intrinsic factor; consequently, the client has pernicious anemia

Nursing Implications/Responsibilities

Procedure:

Step 1

1. An IM injection of B12 is given to saturate all receptor sites for vitamin B12.

2. Client takes a "tagged" oral B12 tablet from nuclear medicine containing a small amount of radioactive material so it can be traced in the client's urine.
3. A 24-hour urine collection is started.
4. After 24 hours, the urine is analyzed. If the "tagged" B12 is found in the urine, pernicious anemia does not exist. The B12 has been absorbed because it has been excreted in the urine. (Remember where urine comes from—the blood). Another reason will have to be diagnosed. Perhaps the client has not had enough B12 in his or her diet. This happens many times with a vegetarian diet.

If no "tagged" B12 is found in the urine, the B12 has not been absorbed into the blood and therefore not excreted in the urine. With this result, a second step is required.

Step 2

1. Another 24-hour urine specimen will be collected following the same steps as above. However, when the "tagged" B12 is given, the intrinsic factor also will be administered.
2. When the urine is analyzed after 24 hours, if the "tagged" B12 is now found in the urine, this means that the B12 has been absorbed and excreted by the kidneys. This would support a diagnosis of pernicious anemia. The intrinsic factor is the deciding factor.

The client with pernicious anemia will be required to take a lifetime monthly dose of B12 either by injection or by nasal spray. With this treatment, anemia will be prevented. Clients usually do quite well.
Education is the key!

Vanillylmandelic Acid Test (VMA Test)

This is a 24-hour urine test, and this lab most likely is ordered to help diagnose a pheochromocytoma or a neuroblastoma. It also can be ordered to evaluate hypertension of unknown origin that has been resistant to standard treatment.

Vanillylmandelic acid is a metabolite of the breakdown of catecholamines (epinephrine and norepinephrine). A pheochromocytoma is a tumor that secretes excess catecholamines outside of the "normal" regulation system. Catecholamines are "normally" released and regulated in conjunction with the sympathetic nervous system, inducing the fight-or-flight response. A pheochromocytoma secretes catecholamines without regard for the sympathetic nervous system, so catecholamines are increased. They are broken down into vanillylmandelic acid as a metabolite, and this is excreted in the urine.

1.4–6.5 mg/24 hr

N/A

N/A

Pheochromocytoma
Neuroblastoma
Ganglioneuroma

If the health-care provider suspects a pheochromocytoma, the client most likely will present with hypertension that fluctuates between extremely high hypertension and normal blood pressure. In other words, the hypertension is intermittent. A tumor secreting catecholamines causes hypertension by constricting blood vessels. The client with a pheochromocytoma also will have other signs and symptoms of the fight-or-flight response since this is a product of catecholamine secretion. The client will have signs and symptoms as follows: increased heart rate, dilated pupils, sweating episodes, and episodes of anxiety and nervousness.

Routine Urinalysis (Dipstick)

Definition/Description

This test is used mainly as a screening test. It screens for infection and liver and kidney problems as well as hydration status. It is usually part of a routine physical.

Urinalysis used as a screening tool is done mainly by a dipstick. The dipstick contains several pads that allow checking for the following items:

- pH
- Protein
- Glucose
- Ketones
- Hemoglobin
- Bilirubin
- Urobilingen
- Nitrate
- Leukocyte esterase
- Specific gravity

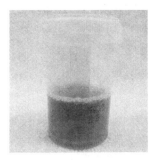

Figure 11-1 Urinalysis

Each of these items will be discussed separately on the following pages.

pH

This part of the urinalysis demonstrates how the kidneys are maintaining the concentration of H^+ ions.

5–9

N/A

Decreased:
Ingestion of cranberries
High-protein diet
Metabolic or respiratory acidosis

Increased:
Ingestion of citrus fruits
Vegetarian diets
Metabolic or respiratory alkalosis

Protein

Definition/Description

As a rule, the presence of protein indicates renal disease, but not 100% of the time.

Less than 20 mg/dL

N/A

N/A

Diabetic nephropathy
Glomerulonephritis
Nephrosis
Toxemia—eclampsia
Benign due to standing, exercise, and stress

Glucose

Definition/Description

This result in urine demonstrates the presence of diabetes. However, this is not a test specifically for diabetes, as the blood glucose has to be very high for the glucose to spill over into the urine.

Normal Result

Negative for glucose

Critical Abnormal Result

Grossly elevated urine glucose needs to be reported, as this indicates very high blood glucose.

Decreased:

N/A

Increased:

Diabetes

Ketones

Definition/Description

The presence of ketones in the urine demonstrates impaired carbohydrate metabolism.

Normal Result

Negative for ketones

Critical Abnormal Result

Ketones, in combination with elevated glucose in the urine, is considered significant and should be reported.

Some Common Reasons for Abnormalities

Decreased:

N/A

Increased:

Diabetes
Starvation
Fasting
Fever
High-protein diet
Vomiting

Hemoglobin

Definition/Description

Hemoglobin in the urine is not normal and could indicate renal disease, the presence of kidney stones, or bladder cancer. These have to be ruled out when hemoglobin is found in the urine.

Normal Result

Negative for hemoglobin

Critical Abnormal Result

N/A

Some Common Reasons for Abnormalities

Decreased:
N/A

Increased:
Malignancy
Glomerulonephritis
Urinary tract infection
Trauma
Exercise
Pyelonephritis
Kidney stone

Bilirubin

Definition/Description

A urine test positive for bilirubin demonstrates the possibility of liver disease.

Negative for bilirubin

N/A

N/A

Cirrhosis
Hepatitis
Tumor in the liver

Urobilingen

Urobilingen can be found in the urine in a very small amount. However, when the amount exceeds the normal amount, the health-care provider should consider the possibility of hepatic or hematopoietic pathology.

Up to 1 mg/dL

N/A

Obstruction of the bile duct

Antibiotic therapy (decreases flora)

Cirrhosis

Hepatitis

Hemolytic anemia

Nitrites

Bacteria in urine convert nitrates to nitrites. Nitrates are found normally in the urine, but the presence of nitrites indicates a urinary tract infection.

Negative for nitrites

N/A

N/A

Presence of nitrite-forming bacteria such as *Klebsiella*, *Proteus*, *Pseudomonas*, *Citrobacter*, *Escherichia*, and some types of *Staphylococcus*

Leukocyte Esterase

Definition/Description

Leukocyte esterase is an enzyme found in neutrophils. In urine, these neutrophils are broken down, and the leukocyte esterase is released. If present in the client's urine, this indicates a urinary tract infection.

Normal Result

Negative for leukocyte esterase

Critical Abnormal Result

N/A

Some Common Reasons for Abnormalities

Decreased:
N/A

Increased:
Bacterial infection
Fungal infection
Parasitic infection
Calculus formation
Glomerulonephritis

Specific Gravity

Definition/Description

This part of the urinalysis demonstrates how well the kidneys are able to concentrate the urine. Many times, with renal failure, the kidneys lose the ability to concentrate urine.

1.001–1.009

N/A

Diabetes insipidus
Excess hydration
Renal failure

Syndrome of inappropriate antidiuretic hormone (SIADH)
Dehydration
Fever
Sweating
Water restriction

Microscopic Urine Examination

A microscopic examination may be indicated in addition to the dipstick urinalysis. Most labs have established criteria for when a microscopic exam is needed.

The microscopic examination assesses the following:

- Red blood cells
- White blood cells
- Renal cells
- Transitional cells
- Squamous cells
- Casts

- Crystals in acid urine
- Crystals in alkaline urine

Bacteria, yeast, or parasites

Each of these items will be discussed separately on the following pages.

Red Blood Cells

Definition/Description

Red blood cells should not be found in the urine in excess of the normal amount of 1–4 hpf. If they occur in greater amounts, many various types of pathology can be indicated.

Normal Result

Less than 5 hpf

Critical Abnormal Result

N/A

Some Common Reasons for Abnormalities

Decreased:
N/A

Increased:
Glomerulonephritis
Calculus
Malignancy
Infection
Trauma

White Blood Cells

Definition/Description

White blood cells should only be found in the urine in very small amounts. If 5 hpf or more are found, some type of pathology is indicated.

Normal Result

Less than 5 hpf

Critical Abnormal Result

N/A

Some Common Reasons for Abnormalities

Decreased:
N/A

Increased:
Urinary tract infection
Nephritis
Fever
Strenuous exercise
Kidney transplant rejection

Renal Cells

Definition/Description

These cells line the collecting ducts and when found in increased amounts in the urine can indicate a variety of pathological conditions.

None

N/A

Decreased:

N/A

Increased:

Acute tubular necrosis
Pyelonephritis
Glomerulonephritis
Malignancy
Drug intoxication
Kidney transplant rejection

Transitional Cells

Definition/Description

These cells line the renal pelvis, ureter, bladder, and urethra but should not be seen in the urine.

Normal Result

None should be seen in the urine.

Critical Abnormal Result

N/A

N/A

Infection

Cancer

Trauma

Squamous Cells

Squamous cells line the vagina and urethra. Normal squamous cells in female urine are of no significance. The presence of abnormal squamous cells requires further examination to rule out cancer.

Rare if found—usually no clinical significance if normal squamous cells are found, especially in the female client.

The presence of abnormal squamous cells in either gender requires further examination.

N/A

N/A

Malignancy

Casts

Casts are tubelike particles that can sometimes be found in microscopic examination of the urine. There are several types of casts such as WBC casts, RBC casts, waxy casts, and hyaline casts. Most types of casts indicate some type of pathology—usually renal. There are some benign causes if hyaline casts are found in the urine. Some of those benign causes can be: fever, exercise, and cold temperatures. However, hyaline casts can indicate non-benign causes also.

Normal Result

No casts should be seen in the urine. On rare occasions, a small amount of hyaline casts can be seen and are there for benign reasons. However, non-benign reasons must be ruled out. Otherwise, no casts should be seen in the urine.

Critical Abnormal Result

N/A

Some Common Reasons for Abnormalities

Possible reasons for casts present:
Acute glomerulonephritis
Subacute bacterial endocarditis
Chronic renal failure
Kidney transplant rejection
Acute pyelonephritis

Crystals in Acid Urine

Definition/Description

Crystals that are found in freshly voided urine are more significant than crystals found in urine that has been standing for two to four hours or more.

Some crystals are all right in small numbers, but it depends on the type of crystal (see below). However, ongoing large numbers found of any crystals in the urine can lead to the formation of stones. The types of crystals that can be found in acid urine are: uric acid, amorphous urates, cystine, cholesterol, and bilirubin.

Cystine, cholesterol, uric acid, and bilirubin crystals are considered abnormal ones with an indication of pathology.

Normal Result

No crystals identified in the urine

Critical Abnormal Result

Presence of the following types of crystals: uric acid, cystine, cholesterol, and bilirubin.
Also, tyrosine and leucine crystals are not necessarily specific to acid urine, but if seen, they usually indicate pathology.

Some Common Reasons for Abnormalities

Cystine crystals: seen in cystinuria
Cholesterol crystals: seen in nephritic syndrome
Bilirubin crystals: seen in liver disease
Uric acid crystals: seen in gout
Tyrosine and leucine crystals: seen in severe liver disease

It is important for the nurse to provide education to the client with a history of crystals in the urine. Stones can develop from ongoing crystals in the urine. Stone formation can depend on the level of hydration, so it is very important to stay well hydrated. It can also depend on the pH of the urine, and this can be altered by the intake of certain foods.

Clients who develop stones are in severe pain, so the nurse must be prepared to administer pain medications. Another major problem for the client experiencing stones is the possibility of obstruction. Consequently, the nurse must be aware of this and constantly assess all components of the urinary/renal system.

Crystals in Alkaline Urine

Definition/Description

Crystals that are found in freshly voided urine are more significant than crystals found in urine that has been standing for two to four hours or more.

Some crystals are non-significant in small numbers; it depends on the type of crystal (see below). However, an ongoing large number of any crystals in the urine can lead to the formation of stones.

The types of crystals that can be found in alkaline urine are: triple phosphate, ammonium biurate, and calcium carbonate. None of these crystals are considered severely pathological such as in tyrosine and leucine crystals. There is always the possibility, however, of stone formation with ongoing crystals in the urine.

Normal Result

No crystals identified in the urine

Critical Abnormal Result

N/A

Triple phosphate: urinary tract infection

Nursing Implications/Responsibilities

It is important for the nurse to provide education to the client with a history of stones. Stone formation can depend on the level of hydration, so it is very important to stay well hydrated. It can also depend on the pH of the urine, and this can be altered by the intake of certain foods.

Clients who experience stones are in severe pain, so the nurse must be prepared to administer pain medications. Another major problem for the client experiencing stones is the possibility of obstruction. In this case, the nurse must be aware of this and constantly assess all components of the urinary/renal system.

Bacteria, Yeast, or Parasites

Definition/Description

Bacteria and yeast may be contaminants or true pathogens. The health-care provider must look at the quantity on the report and then assess the client's signs and symptoms. The provider must also consider how the specimen was obtained. Another specimen by a different collection method may be indicated as well as cultures. Parasites should not be present in the urine.

Normal Result

Negative: No identification of bacteria, yeast, or parasites

Critical Abnormal Result

N/A

Some Common Reasons for Abnormalities

Increased:
Urinary tract infection

Image credit

- Fig. 11.1: Copyright © James Heilman, MD (CC BY-SA 3.0) at https://commons.wikimedia.org/wiki/File%3ARhabdoUrine.JPG.

12 CEREBROSPINAL FLUID (CSF) LABS

CSF Analysis

Pressure

Definition/Description

Pressure is measured during a spinal tap. It should be less than 20 cm H_2O. An increased pressure above this is indicative of bleeding, infection, or tumors.

Normal Result

Less than 20 cm H_2O

Nursing Implications/Responsibilities

For an accurate measurement, the client should be in a lateral recumbent position. The client should be told to relax as much as possible when the pressure readings are taken.

Color and Appearance

Definition/Description

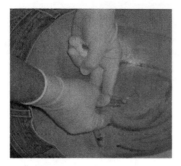

Figure 12-1 Getting a Lumbar Puncture.

Cerebrospinal fluid (CSF) should be clear and colorless. If it is hazy, this could indicate that the cell count is elevated, which could indicate a variety of conditions such as infection. If it is red, pink, or orange, this could indicate the presence of red blood cells. A yellow color could indicate the presence of bilirubin, which could mean increased breakdown of red blood cells or subarachnoid hemorrhage.

Normal Result

Clear and colorless

Cells

Definition/Description

Increased cells in cerebrospinal fluid can be an indication of infection, a tumor, or blood. As indicated below, a few cells are normal, but an increased amount is not.

Normal Result

0–5 small lymphocytes/mm^3

Protein

Definition/Description

As noted below, a certain amount of protein is normal in cerebrospinal fluid. Decreased or increased amounts can indicate pathology. A viral infection is suspected with a protein count of 50–200 mg/dL, whereas a bacterial infection has a higher protein count, usually 500 mg/dL or more. Guillain-Barre syndrome and encephalitis also can present with increased protein. Hyperthyroidism can present with decreased protein.

Normal Result

Adult: 15–45 mg/dL
Older adult: 15–60 mg/dL

Glucose

Definition/Description

As can be seen below, a certain amount of glucose is normal in cerebrospinal fluid. But a decreased amount below normal is usually indicative of some type of infection. Remember, organisms like to feed on glucose, so it will be decreased! Decreased glucose levels can be suggestive of bacterial, viral, or fungal meningitis. Leukemia and other cancers also present with decreased glucose levels in the CSF.

Normal Result

40–70 mg/dL or 60–70% of client's current blood glucose level

Critical Abnormal Result

Less than 37 mg/dL
Greater than 440 mg/dL

Lactic Acid

Increased amounts of lactic acid in the CSF indicate cerebral hypoxia with anaerobic metabolism. This can occur with bacterial, fungal, or tubercular meningitis.

Less than 25.2mg/dL

IgG

This is one of the most important proteins. Its presence in excess can indicate some type of autoimmune or inflammatory process such as multiple sclerosis, neurosyphilis, or a viral infection.

Less than 3.4 mg/dL

Gram Stain

A Gram stain can be either positive or negative. If it is positive, the organisms take on a dark purple stain under the microscope. Gram-negative organisms take on a pink color under the microscope.

Some of the Gram-positive organisms are *Staphylococcus*, *Streptococcus*, *Clostridium*, *Enterococcus*, and *Bacillus*.

Some of the Gram-negative organisms are *Enterobacter, Escherichia, Neisseria, Proteus, Salmonella, Aeromonas, and Campylobacter.*

Normal Result

Negative

Critical Abnormal Result

Positive Gram stain, India ink preparation, or culture

Nursing Implications/Responsibilities

Some of the organisms may require some type of isolation. You should notify infection control and refer to the isolation procedures at your facility.

Image credit

- Fig. 12.1: Copyright © Brainhell (CC BY-SA 3.0) at https://commons. wikimedia.org/wiki/File%3AWikipedian_getting_a_lumbar_puncture_(2006).jpg.

REFERENCES

Ignatavicius, D.D., & Workman, M.L. (2016). *Medical-surgical nursing: Patient-centered collaborative care* (8th ed). St. Louis, MO: Elsevier.

Van Leeuwen, A.M, & Bladh, M.L. (2015). *Davis's comprehensive handbook of laboratory and diagnostic tests* (6th ed). Philadelphia, PA: F.A. Davis Company.

NOTES

INDEX

Labs Listed Alphabetically

CPSIA information can be obtained
at www.ICGtesting.com
Printed in the USA
LVOW10s2038010118
561452LV00011B/49/P